The Power of Auras

Tap Into Your Energy Field for Clarity, Peace of Mind, and Well-Being

Susan Shumsky, DD

New Page BOOKS

A Division of The Career Press, Inc.
Pompton Plains, NJ

The Power of Auras
Edited by Kirsten Dalley
Typeset by Gina Talucci
Cover design by Lucia Rossman/Digi Dog Design
Printed in the U.S.A.

To order this title, please call toll-free 1-800-CAREER-1 (NJ and Canada: 201-848-0310) to order using VISA or MasterCard, or for further information on books from Career Press.

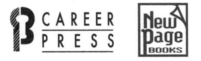

The Career Press, Inc.
220 West Parkway, Unit 12
Pompton Plains, NJ 07444
www.careerpress.com
www.newpagebooks.com

Library of Congress Cataloging-in-Publication Data
CIP Data Available Upon Request.

The Power of Auras can familiarize readers with the complex subject of the human energy field, spiritual healing, affirmation, and yoga, but it in no way claims to fully teach the techniques described. Therefore, personal instruction is recommended.

The Power of Auras is not an independent guide for self-healing. Susan Shumsky is not a medical doctor, psychiatrist, or psychologist, and she does not diagnose diseases or prescribe treatments. No medical claims or cures are implied in this book, even if specific "benefits," "healing," or "treatments" are mentioned. Readers are advised to practice the methods in this book only with the permission of a qualified medical doctor or psychiatrist, and to use these methods at their own risk.

Susan Shumsky, Divine Revelation®, Teaching of Intuitional Metaphysics, New Page Books, and any other affiliate, agent, assign, licensee, and authorized representatives make no claim or obligation and take no legal responsibility for the effectiveness, results, or benefits of reading this book or of using the suggested methods; deny all liability for any injuries or damages that readers may incur; and are to be held harmless against any claim, liability, loss, or damage caused by or arising from following any suggestions made in this book or from contacting anyone listed in this book or at *www.divinerevelation.org*.

All of the testimonials in this book are real, but some names, occupations, or places of residence have been changed.

This book is dedicated to our beloved
Rich Bell and Peter Meyer,
who have departed to their heavenly abode.
Their wisdom, loving kindness, and care inspired these powerful
teachings of cleansing, healing, and lifting the human and
atmospheric energy fields.

Acknowledgments

ॐ

Many people have generously contributed their love, energy, and wisdom to this book. First, I want to thank our beloved departed Peter Meyer, my wonderful mentor on this path. Also, our dearly departed Rich Bell, with love, for the inspiration of his magnificent healing prayers. I also thank Connie Huebner for offering her profound prayers. I thank Joey Korn for his incredible research into vortices and grids. I am grateful to Gladys McCoy, Thomas Milliren, Tony Gehringer, Joan McFarlane, Carl Bracy, and Walt Woods, all of whom have shared their amazing experiences. I also want to thank all other master dowsers with whom I have had the privilege to study.

I thank all the staff at Career Press/New Page Books, especially Michael Pye. Thank you, Michael, for bringing out a new edition of this book. I also want to thank Gina Talucci, Laurie Kelly-Pye, Adam Schwartz, and my editor, Kirsten Dalley.

But mostly, I want to thank my agents, Jeff and Deborah Herman, for standing by me so many years and never giving up.

Contents

ఇం

Part III: Cleansing Your Energy Field

Part IV: Strengthening Your Energy Field

Foreword

ಲಚಿ

By Dannion Brinkley

When I had my first near-death experience in 1975, my soul lifted out of my physical body and I found myself high above my body. Hovering just below the ceiling of my bedroom, I watched as my family and friends tried desperately to resuscitate me. In those critical moments, I caught my first glimpse of the human energy field, or light-body. This aura surrounds all living beings, and it displays radiant, multifaceted, jewel-like, and prismatic hues and tones.

In my out-of-body state, I witnessed the fact that our auras actually change in color and intensity, according to the changing of our moods. As my loved ones struggled to revive me, their auras would spike sharply, with shades of deep red and orange, as they experienced feelings of frustration and despair. As I traveled down the tunnel and into the Light, I continued to be fascinated by the fluid nature and breathtaking beauty of the other light-bodies I encountered along the way.

Of course, within the Crystal City, I beheld the most magnificent sight of all. The Thirteen Beings of Light who welcomed me at the Hall of Knowledge were more glorious and brilliant than anything one could ever imagine. Thinking back, I now realize that the Beings of Light on the other side were so exquisitely luminous because, as we grow spiritually and advance in our capacity to love unconditionally, our aura intensifies and expands in direct proportion. Knowing this firsthand, it was with great interest that I read Dr. Shumsky's book. Having studied it from cover to cover, there is now no doubt in my mind that she has captured the spiritual truth and essence of the human aura.

Dr. Susan Shumsky is one of the most genuine, sincere spiritual teachers that I am privileged to personally know. She is a rare treasure who truly walks her talk, and her profound connection with inner divinity is obvious. Her integrity and wisdom shine forth in this amazing book, which helps anyone to see and feel subtle energy and to heal blockages in their energy field. The affirmations and prayers offered in this book can transform your life. Use them now, and discover peace of mind, well-being, joy, mental clarity, self-authority, and inner strength.

Dannion Brinkley
Author, *Saved by the Light*

Introduction

ಌ

This planet is undergoing a dramatic spiritual transition. As a result, many people are feeling lost. You can no longer depend on institutions you counted on in the past. As old patterns crumble, a new way of life will test your ability to rely on yourself as never before. The old ways are gone, and in this new world, you will determine your own fate and walk a unique path that is right for you. No longer can you just follow the norm while daydreaming that governments, employers, or any other agent will provide safety. There are no guarantees, as job security, pensions, investments, and savings are dwindling, and many people grow increasingly fearful.

In this atmosphere of uncertainty, one thing is sure: The self-reliant and self-sufficient will thrive, and you must be adaptable to this radically changing world if you want to survive. At this time, as never before, it is imperative to gain and maintain inner stability and strength. That is why it is timely for a new edition of this book, formerly titled *Exploring Auras*, to be issued.

This highly acclaimed, positively reviewed, greatly respected book has helped countless readers learn how to use powerful methods of spiritual healing in order to gain greater inner strength, become more self-reliant, and attain and maintain self-integrity. Thousands of people have found the book invaluable—especially those in the holistic health field who use these methods for clients in their daily practice. With a different name and cover and several improvements, this new edition, *The Power of Auras*, will bring the message of self-authority and self-sufficiency to even more people who desperately need greater strength during this time of change.

What do auras have to do with self-reliance? You will discover the answer as you learn the methods in this book, which will help you cleanse your energy field, increase its strength and charisma, and keep it clear, bright, and sparkling with life-force energy.

My Experience of Auras

The first time I remember seeing an aura was in junior high school. My highly eccentric math teacher, the fabulous Mr. Niederhut, often climbed up onto his desk and squatted like a bird perched on a tree limb. From his vantage, I imagine he could more easily access the heights of algebra, set theory, and all the other mathematical esoteria that inspired his students so deeply.

Mr. Niederhut had a big aura. I could see energy around his head, and the radiations of that energy moved and vibrated around him. However, at age 14, in 1962, I can say with certainty that not one person I knew had a clue what an aura was.

Happily, however, a few years later my friend Bev began to open my eyes to subtle energies. And, due to her influence, I soared into an adventure that led me from the hippie havens of Haight-Ashbury to the heights of the Himalayas in India, where I studied in the ashram of Maharishi Mahesh Yogi, famous guru of the Beatles and of Deepak Chopra. I remained in Maharishi's ashram for 22 years, and I served on his personal staff for seven of those years.

During my ashram years, I meditated up to 20 hours a day. Sometimes I went into my room and did not appear for up to eight weeks at a time. Food was brought to my door. I practiced silence and never uttered a sound for up to four months at a time. I fasted for up to two months at a time. I practiced complete celibacy.

After spending 22 years with my eyes closed, I finally discovered something I had sought for lifetimes but did not find in ashram life. I discovered how to listen to the "still small voice" of God within, how to have direct divine communication and contact. Peter Meyer of San Diego, founder of Teaching of Intuitional Metaphysics, helped me develop ESP—extrasensory perception, the "sixth sense" used to perceive, feel, sense, and see auras.

In this book you will learn some of the skills that helped me develop my subtle sensory perception, and you will practice methods that can enhance your own.

What You Will Learn Here

In this book you will learn everything you ever wanted to know about the subtle energy field, and how to see it, sense it, measure it, clear it, strengthen it, and enhance it. This book will help you master many disciplines that can increase the energy to your field, disciplines that include subtle sense perception, spiritual healing, intuitive kinesiology, color and sound therapy, breathing, movement, meditation, affirmative prayer, and visualization.

By using the easy-to-learn, proven, time-tested tools and techniques presented here, you can receive the following benefits:

- *Develop subtle sensory perception to see or sense auras.* Mary Albertson, a psychologist from Vancouver, Washington, states: "I always thought that to see auras I would have to see shapes of color around a person's head. Now I realize that I can perceive auras by seeing or feeling them with my eyes closed. This new skill has been very helpful in my counseling practice."

- *Overcome psychic sponge syndrome, oversensitivity, and psychic vampirism.* "I was one of those psychic sponges like Susan talked about in her workshop," reports Nel Krafi, a teacher from Fort Worth, Texas. "Since I started using her techniques for keeping my aura closed off to all but my higher self, I feel more inwardly directed, more grounded, and less influenced by people who think they know better what is right for me than I do."

§ *Develop spiritual self-defense, auric protection, and self-reliance.* Elliot Atkins, an accountant from Denver, Colorado, writes, "Thank you so much for your books. I have read many, many books, from Deepak to Gawain and then some, and your books are by far the most complete, informative and important. I especially like your points about 'protection.' I think that more people need to know about this."

§ *Increase power, balance, focus, and clarity in your energy field.* Rose Ellerbie, a mother from Levittown, Pennsylvania, reports, "My life and mind were in disarray before I learned how to heal my energy body and keep myself free of influences from other people. I found a peaceful centeredness that I never experienced before. Thank you, Susan, for your wonderful centering and grounding techniques."

§ *Heal and release dense vibrations in your environment.* "At a trade show I took Dr. Shumsky's workshop 'How to Raise the Spiritual Vibrations in Your Store,' says Jonah Rathford, a bookstore owner from Omaha, Nebraska. "I put this into practice and cleared the astral cobwebs inhabiting my space. The store took on a brightness that has attracted more customers, who often comment on what good vibrations it has."

§ *Release attachments and addictions crystallized in your energy field.* Jacob Radolfsky, a salesman from Hoboken, New Jersey, states, "Since using the prayers in Susan Shumsky's book, I now have hope. I thought that I was lost and would never find a way out. I have been battling alcoholism for several years, and I felt helpless. These prayers have helped me become strong enough to join AA and to stick with the program."

§ *Cut psychic ties and cords to create healthier relationships.* Russell Valkenberg, a builder from Memphis, Tennessee, states, "The affirmations that we learned in Susan Shumsky's workshop have had a powerful, positive effect on how I see myself in relationship to my family, friends, and coworkers. Now I feel less anxious about how people see me."

   ॐ   *Overcome psychic nets, clamps, shackles, plates, hooks, tentacles, arrows, jails, holes, leaks, armors, masks, shells, entities, environmental static, and geopathic zones.* A massage therapist from Bakersfield, California, Veronica Lott, says, "Since using the healing prayers that Susan taught at our church, I am amazed at how effective these simple affirmations are. I use them for my clients when I see anomalies in their energy field, and the results are spectacular. I want to express how these healing prayers have changed my life."

   ॐ   *Heal and augment human and environmental energy fields.* Stephanie McMullin, a hairdresser from Milwaukee, Wisconsin, says, "Your healing techniques have had a dramatic effect on the health of my aura and my surroundings. They are so simple to practice that even I can do them. I feel a difference in my own life and in my home, work, and everywhere that I focus on to use the techniques. Thank you for this gift, Dr. Shumsky. You are a blessing to the earth."

What Is in This Book

The Power of Auras is arranged into four parts:

   ॐ   Part I introduces the human energy field (aura) and explains how it brings life to individuals. Chapter 1 describes the aura and how you will benefit by learning more about it. Chapter 2 explores *prana*, the vital principle that gives life to your energy field. Chapter 3 provides a roadmap to your inner life, levels of the subtle body, and planes of existence. Chapter 4 describes the most exciting research about the subtle body and energy field.

   ॐ   Part II helps you see, feel, and experience subtle energy through several different methods. Chapter 5 gives specific exercises to help you develop your clairvoyant sight and clairsentient feeling of auras. In Chapter 6 you learn to use tools, such as pendulums and L-rods, to measure the aura. In Chapter 7 you discover how clairvoyants see auras and thought-forms.

In Chapter 8 you learn to interpret the meaning of colors you see in the aura.

    ॐ Part III helps you heal not only your own auric field, but also energy fields in your surroundings. In Chapter 9 you heal and transmute dense environmental energies, including astral influences and environ-mental static. In Chapter 10 you ground and protect your auric field, and become less affected by environmental influences. In Chapter 11 you heal your mental body, thought-forms, and negative emotions. Chapter 12 offers profound prayers that heal and lift your aura.

    ॐ Part IV teaches methods for augmenting and enhancing your energy field. In Chapter 13 you use color and sound to vitalize the subtle energy field and rejuvenate the physical body. In Chapter 14 you practice easy yogic breathing methods that brighten and expand your aura. In Chapter 15 you use simple, powerful exercises with immediate, profound results that invigorate your energy field. Chapter 16 helps you use tools to strengthen the human energy field and heal geopathic energy zones. In Chapter 17 you practice meditation to lift, strengthen, expand, and energize your subtle body and auric field.

How This Book Can Transform You

You might be delighted, uplifted, or challenged by this book. I guarantee, however, that you will be transformed, if you are willing to practice the simple methods offered here. These techniques are so easy that anyone can do them. All that is required is a willingness to participate.

You can change your life, beginning today. You can let go of the mental, emotional, and energetic blocks you have carried in your energy field. These blocks no longer serve you. Release them now. You can become free, clear, and joyous. Now that you have discovered what this book has to offer, let us begin a powerful journey together—a voyage that will lift your spirit, free your mind, heal your body, and make your soul sing. It is said that the journey of a thousand miles begins with one step.

Let us take that step together now.

Part I

⚜

Discovering Your Energy Field

1

What's an Aura, Anyway?

ನಾ

Introducing Energy Fields

"He who stays with the sun will know no darkness."
—Nisargadatta[1]

During my travels I met Jodie, a massage therapist from Dallas, who had studied and practiced spiritual healing for decades. During a private session with Jodie, I perceived with my inner eye a bizarre anomaly in her energy field: It looked like a large, thick, rectangular sheet of armor in front of her face and upper torso. I called this a "psychic plate," and it had been installed in her aura by a so-called spiritual teacher named Kriya, whom Jodie considered to be a highly evolved spiritual master. After I used a healing affirmation to dissolve the plate, Jodie asked me whether it was wise for her to continue studying with Kriya. My reply was, "If you enjoy having a psychic

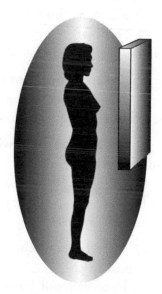

Figure 1a. Psychic Plate

plate in front of your face so you cannot see the truth, so you cannot hear the divine voice, and so you cannot feel love, then, by all means, continue to follow Kriya."

This story illustrates a simple point. We all have misconceptions about the human energy field, no matter how long we have studied or practiced spiritual healing. And we can all be duped by teachers whom we consider to be more highly evolved than we are.

Therefore, let us begin with some basics and answer a few of your questions.

FAQs About Experiences of Subtle Energy

Q: **"I am not clairvoyant. How can I learn to read auras?"**

A: This book offers many simple tools and techniques to help you read auras without any special abilities. Here you will also learn to develop subtle sensory perception so you can begin to feel, sense, or see auras.

Q: **"Do I have healing abilities, and can I start a healing practice?"**

A: Everyone has healing abilities that can be developed. In this book you will learn many methods for healing your own energy field and that of others. Most of these techniques require no previous abilities or training.

Q: **"What can I do about being controlled by other people and getting drained, as though vampires are sapping my energy?"**

A: This book provides ways to overcome what I call *psychic sponge syndrome*—oversensitivity to environmental influences.

Q: **"I experience a lot of fear. How can I overcome this?"**

A: This book helps you develop spiritual self-defense and experience the safety, security, and protection of your higher self.

Q: **"What can I do when I feel off-balance, scattered, confused, and ineffective?"**

A: Using simple methods that anyone can do, you will learn, through this book, how to be more powerful, centered, balanced, focused, and clear in your energy field.

Q: **"I feel overwhelmed by negative thoughts and emotions. Can I move past this?"**

A: Here you will learn and practice specific healing affirmations and prayers that help you transform and transmute your mental/emotional body.

Q: **"How can I handle the creepy vibes in my office?"**

A: This book will help you heal and release the dense vibrations in your environmental atmosphere.

Q: **"How can I have better relationships at home and at work?"**

A: Here you will use techniques and tools for working with subtle energy fields to create healthier relationships.

Q: **"Can I overcome the havoc that codependency and addiction have wreaked?"**

A: In this book you will learn to release undue attachments and addictions that have become crystallized in your energy field.

Q: **"Is this easy to practice? Or do I have to struggle with difficult, strict, hard-to-follow disciplines?"**

A: This book is easy to understand, logical, and practical, with simple-to-learn methods requiring no previous experience, background, training, or knowledge.

Take the Aura IQ Test

Okay, calling all experts to test your "Aura IQ." Maybe you have studied spiritual healing for decades, and you believe that you are an authority on the subject. Perhaps you think this book is too elementary for you. Even if you think you are an expert, the following test just might stump you.

1. What does the word *aura* mean?
    A. A sphere of energy.
    B. A bubble of protection.
    C. A breeze.
    D. A circle around the body.
    E. A chocolate cookie sandwich with cream filling.

2. What is the human energy field?
    A. A place from which we receive energy.
    B. A higher plane of existence.
    C. Higher consciousness.
    D. The subtle bodies.
    E. Where to get drinks that give you a buzz for five hours.

3. What does the word *prana* mean?
   A. Moving or breathing forth.
   B. Subtle energy.
   C. The breath of life.
   D. A breathing exercise.
   E. A man-eating fish.

4. What is a thought-form?
   A. A negative idea, habit, or condition.
   B. A strong belief or idea that has crystallized.
   C. The mental body.
   D. The subconscious mind.
   E. A fantasy about Kate Beckinsale.

5. What is a power spot?
   A. A place where energy leys intersect.
   B. A place where powerful entities reside.
   C. An earth energy grid.
   D. A crop circle.
   E. A dog in a detergent commercial.

6. What is a psychic tie?
   A. A spiritual connection.
   B. A love connection.
   C. A binding attachment.
   D. A rope, string, or cord.
   E. Houdini's straitjacket.

7. What is a façade body?
   A. A mask that hides your true self.
   B. A subtle body that embodies your higher self.
   C. A thought-form in your intellect.
   D. A subtle body that embodies your mind.
   E. Marilyn Manson dressed up as Alice Cooper.

8. What is the food sheath?
   A. The physical body.
   B. The astral body.

C. The mental body.

D. The subtle body.

E. A muzzle you wear to prevent overeating.

9. What is the mental body?

    A. A subtle body made of crystallized thoughts.

    B. A subtle body made of the higher mind.

    C. The ego and intellect.

    D. The *atman*.

    E. A suit that Ironman wears.

10. What is the blissful sheath?

    A. A subtle body made of the higher self.

    B. The causal body.

    C. The higher mental body.

    D. The veil that covers your true mental body.

    E. Something you find in your brother's wallet.

11. What does the word *chakra* mean?

    A. A wheel.

    B. The center of the body.

    C. When it opens, you become enlightened.

    D. A nerve ending.

    E. That awful screeching blackboard sound.

12. What does the word *kundalini* mean?

    A. A goddess from India.

    B. Curled-up energy.

    C. A sign that you are experiencing higher consciousness.

    D. A snake or serpent.

    E. A pasta.

13. What is an astral entity?

    A. A person who died.

    B. An evil spirit.

    C. An earthbound spirit.

    D. A higher being who gives information through channeling.

    E. A baseball player for the Houston team.

14. What is muscle-testing?
    A. A way to heal astral entities.
    B. A way to heal your body.
    C. A way to enhance your energy field.
    D. A way to measure the weakness or strength of your muscles.
    E. Something they do on a beach in Venice, California.

15. What is a psychic sponge?
    A. An overly sensitive person.
    B. Someone with psychic abilities.
    C. A psychic vampire.
    D. A negative person.
    E. Something used to mop up your psyche.

16. What is clairsentience?
    A. Clear seeing.
    B. Clear sound.
    C. Clear sensing.
    D. Clear scent.
    E. Clair de Lune's twin sister.

17. What can mirror gazing do?
    A. Help you develop clairvoyance.
    B. Help you hear the inner voice.
    C. Help you get the answer to a question.
    D. Help you read minds.
    E. Tell you who's the fairest of them all.

18. What is an L-rod?
    A. A tool used by psychics to tell the future.
    B. A tool that drills for water.
    C. A tool that surpasses your intuition.
    D. An angle rod or swing rod.
    E. The founder of the Church of Scientology.

19. What is a pendulum?
    A. Something that counts time.
    B. A weight attached to an armature.
    C. A crystal hanging from a chain.

D. A tool that predicts the future.

E. A scary book by Edgar Allen Poe.

20. What is kinesiology?

    A. The study of movement.

    B. Muscle-testing.

    C. Telepathy.

    D. Dowsing.

    E. A wrestling match with your chiropractor.

Scoring Your Test

Here you can place a check mark to the left of those answers that you answered correctly. The answers to this test are as follows:

1. C. The word *aura* derives from ancient Greek for "breath of air" or "breeze": *avra*.

2. D. The human energy field consists of subtle bodies that permeate and surround the physical body.

3. A. The Sanskrit word *prana* means "moving or breathing forth."

4. B. A thought-form is an idea or concept with so much intensity of energy that it crystallizes and takes a subtle structure.

5. A. A power spot is a place with powerful, aura-strengthening earth energies where energy leys intersect.

6. C. A psychic tie is an undue attachment or repulsion to any person, place, thing, organization, situation, circumstance, memory, experience, or addiction.

7. A. A façade body is a mask or veil that you wear, a false persona that you project, which hides who you really are.

8. A. The food sheath is the physical body, which is created and sustained by food, and which becomes food for something else after death.

9. A. The mental body consists of thought-forms—crystallized thoughts and emotions.

10. B. The blissful sheath consists of the causal body—progenitor of individual ego.

11. A. The Sanskrit word *chakra* means "wheel," because its hub links many conduits of subtle energy, and its spokes radiate subtle energy.

12. B. The Sanskrit root *kundal* means "curled up." *Kundalini* is a special spiritual energy coiled at the base of the spine.

13. C. An astral entity is often a soul, who, for various reasons, did not go into the divine light after death and is therefore "earthbound."

14. Muscle-testing shows whether your muscles are weakened or strengthened. This can test how your energy field is affected by various influences.

15. A. A psychic sponge is a person who absorbs vibrations from the environment as a sponge absorbs water.

16. C. Clairsentience is a French term meaning "clear feeling."

17. A. Mirror gazing is a practice that helps develop clairvoyant sight ("clear seeing" in English).

18. D. An L-rod, also called angle rod or swing rod, can be used to find lost objects, measure invisible energies, and enhance your intuition.

19. B. A pendulum is a device with a weight attached to an armature (usually a string or chain). It can be used to measure subtle energy.

20. A. *Kinesis* means "movement," and *-ology* means "science or branch of knowledge." So *kinesiology* means "the study of movement."

Evaluating Your Test

⚹ If you got 20 right, congratulations! Your Aura IQ is 200. With a perfect score, you are titled Doctor of Aura Power.

⚹ If you got 15–19 right, you are a Master of Aura Power. You have delved deeply into spiritual studies, and your Aura IQ is 175.

⚹ If you got 10–14 right, you are a Bachelor of Aura Power. You know a lot, but you have a few things to learn. Your Aura IQ is 150.

- ♨ If you got 5–9 right, this book will be an eye-opener. You will learn much here. Your Aura IQ is 125.

- ♨ If you got 1–4 right, the odds are with you. You have successfully proven that random selection works. Your Aura IQ is 100.

- ♨ If you got them all wrong, I would not be surprised. Your Aura IQ is 75.

- ♨ If you chose any E's, congratulations. At least you have a sense of humor.

Are you surprised at some of the answers on the test? If so, it's because many myths surround the terms mentioned there. Having some familiarity with these esoteric terms is not the same as understanding them deeply. In this book you will gain profound understanding of all these terms, and you will learn how to use them in everyday, practical life to enhance your energy field. Let us begin now with an in-depth answer to Question 1 on the Aura IQ Test.

What Does the Word "Aura" Mean?

Have you ever wondered, *What is keeping my body alive? What energy gives life to my body with my first breath, and what energy will leave my body when I die?*

Let us consider some fundamental questions. Obviously you have a physical body, which seems to run by itself: Lungs breathe, food digests, and blood rushes through your veins. Yet what makes it breathe? What makes your heart beat continually? What keeps it running like a clock, and what makes it stop? The answers to these questions seem elusive.

No medical doctor can tell you why, with a baby's first cry, the miracle of life begins, or why, with the last rasp of death, this same miracle comes to an end. Although a doctor can describe all the systems of your body and how they function, no one has unveiled the true secret of life.

However, as we look to the Far East, we can begin to unlock this mystery. The ancients of India and China discovered a precious, invisible, imperceptible substance that animates your body and, indeed, bestows life on the cosmos. This precious life essence, called *prana,* is that fundamental energy. In this book you will discover this *pranic energy*, or life-force, and you will learn how to strengthen that power in your life.

Your physical body is not the only body you inhabit. You also have a subtle body, consisting of several layers, or sheaths. Your subtle body, which pervades and surrounds your physical body, is called your *energy field*, or *aura*. For most people, the subtle body is invisible, both to the eye and to nearly all scientific measuring instruments.

In the ancient Sanskrit language the root *ar* means "spoke of a wheel," indicating that the aura radiates from the body as the spokes of a wheel radiate from the hub. The ancient Greek word *avra* means "breath of air" or "breeze"—the vital energy that breathes life into your being. So the subtle energy field, which permeates and envelops your body, is your *auric field*—a multifaceted, multidimensional sphere of immense light, power, and vitality.

The breath of air that gives you life also breathes life into the cosmos. Thus everything in the universe is filled and surrounded by auric fields that you can experience, measure, evaluate, cleanse, heal, restore, and strengthen.

This book will help you increase your own pranic energy and augment the energy in your surroundings through simple yet powerful methods that produce profound results instantaneously. Here you will not only discover auric fields; you will also cleanse and strengthen your own aura and the auras of others. Indeed, you will master the art of healing the energy field of your environment, home, workplace, city, nation—even your planet.

Are you ready to begin your adventure to unlock the power of auras? Are you willing to become an inner-space explorer and discover who you really are? Are you ready to unearth mysterious realms of invisible, secret, unexplored places? Now is time to dive into the unknown depths of your heart and find the treasures buried within.

Let us get started now!

2

How Bright Is Your Aura?

ᴓᴓ

Discovering Pranic Energies

"A candle never loses anything when it lights another candle."
—Anonymous[1]

Have you ever met a person who had a powerful, wonderful vibration? Someone you wanted to get closer to? Have you met another person whose vibration gave you the creeps? Can you tell immediately whether you will like someone—or not? Have you ever felt someone was standing too close, and you had to step back?

If you answered yes to any of these questions, you have experienced a subtle energy that pervades every individual and affects people in profound ways. In this chapter we will explore the mysteries of this subtle energy—*prana*.

Life-Force Energy

The Sanskrit word *prana*, not readily translatable into English, derives from roots *pra* ("first," "primary," "before," or "forth") and *an* ("breathe," "move," "live"). So *prana* means "moving or breathing forth." However, prana is much more than breath. It is cosmic energy, sometimes called *absolute energy*, which gives life to all matter in the universe.

Prana is the power within all things and all beings, from elementary quantum particles to complex life forms. As the finest vital force in everything, prana manifests on the physical plane as motion and on the mental plane as thought.

Prana is in the air, yet it is not oxygen or any other physical constituent of air. All living things absorb prana with every breath. Yet, if prana were absent from air, no organism could survive by breathing air. Prana is in every particle of creation, but is not a particle.

The *élan vital*, or vital life energy, of prana is called *chi* or *qi* in China, and *ki* in Japan. The Chinese practice of Qigong uses qi for healing. In ancient Egypt *ka* was the force linking the body to the spiritual world. In fact, 97 world cultures have names for pranic energy, according to John White in his book *Future Science*.

In the Bible's book of Genesis, the Hebrew term *neshemet ruach chayim* is translated as "breath of life." The word *neshemet* means "ordinary breath found in the air." *Chayim* means "life." But the word *ruach* means the "spirit of life," which refers to pranic energy.

> *"And the LORD God formed man of the dust of the ground, and breathed into his nostrils the breath of life; and man became a living soul."*[2]

Western science completely denies the existence of prana, which is, indeed, life itself. That is because prana is a non-material substance, not measurable by any instrument. It pervades all of creation and penetrates areas where air cannot reach.

So what is this mysterious substance or prana that is entirely without substance?

Prana Is Life Itself

Prana is key to all life in the universe. Your body is alive by virtue of prana. It is responsible for heartbeat, breathing, digestion, and excretion. Pranic currents produce movement of eyelids, walking, playing, running, talking, thinking, reasoning, feeling, and willing. Pranic energy manufactures semen, gastric juice, bile, intestinal juice, and saliva.

Both oxygen and prana are required to keep you alive. Oxygen in the air flows through your circulatory system to build and replenish your blood.

Prana in the air moves through your nervous system to bring strength and energy. Prana resembles electric currents flowing through your body, transmitting commands from your brain through your nerves.

Without prana, you would be a corpse. You could not move or breathe. Your blood would not circulate, lungs would not move, and body would be stiff and cold. It is said in the ancient Hatha Yoga Pradipika of India, "When there is prana in the body it is called life; when it leaves the body it results in death."[3]

Your vital body, through which prana flows, is attached to your physical body at the navel through a thread-sized pranic link. When this link is severed, prana is cut off. Your vital and physical bodies then separate, and death occurs. The enormous pranic energy keeping your physical body alive then withdraws into your subtle body.

Using Prana to Your Advantage

Your aura is made of prana. Intensifying pranic energy increases vitality, health, power, influence, charisma, willpower, and supernormal powers. The spiritual power within you can be awakened by using prana consciously.

Pranic energy is continually drained by every thought, word, and deed, and is consistently replenished by every breath. Other sources of prana are sunlight, water, air, and food. Prana is soaked up by skin from fresh air, bathing, swimming, and sunbathing. It is inhaled into the nostrils and lungs. *Food-prana* is imbibed through your tongue, mouth, and teeth and the action of your saliva, as you masticate nutritious food. *Water-prana* is absorbed by bathing, swimming, and by drinking refreshing, pure water.

Thought is the most refined, potent form of prana. Therefore, when thoughts become more refined and spiritually attuned, pranic energy increases. When your mind is relaxed and expanded during deep meditation, pranic energy is boosted exponentially.

Speech vibrates with pranic energy, and certain forms of speech, such as prayer and affirmation, increase pranic energy. Positive, powerful statements of truth expand your aura. But negative, damaging, harmful speech diminishes and shrinks your aura.

A vibrant, large, expanded, bright, smooth, elegant, energetic aura surrounds a healthy individual with abundant pranic energy. A small, contracted, dark, dingy, stifled, lethargic, jagged, sluggish aura surrounds a person who is ill, depressed, depleted, or emotionally distressed.

How bright is your aura? Do you want to enhance or expand it? You can imbibe more prana and thereby bring greater vitality to your aura. This book offers powerful, positive methods specifically designed to increase the size, intensity, and health of your energy field.

Conserving Pranic Energy

Pranic energy is used by everyone. When you need to lift a heavy object, solve a complex problem, or overcome danger, your first impulse is to hold your breath. This draws on an extra supply of prana to accomplish the task. If you are injured, you unconsciously hold your breath and then touch the injured part of your body. Thereby, pranic energy is transferred through your touch. Your instincts know about prana, even if your mind does not.

When you inhale, prana enters your body and is stored in your subtle energy centers. The more pranic energy you absorb, the more healing and vitality rushes to every cell. Yogic breathing methods (*pranayama*) collect and conserve pranic energy in your solar plexus, your pranic storage battery. Yogic breathing saturates your physical body with pranic energy, preventing disease and augmenting willpower, concentration, self-control, and spiritual awakening.

Moderate exercise, such as walking, bicycling, swimming, and yoga exercises (*asanas*), along with proper breathing and *pranayama,* oxygenates blood and revitalizes vital energy—without the strain or oxygen debt of heavy exercise.

Deep meditation automatically controls breathing, which becomes slow, regular, and quiet. In the state of *samadhi* (equanimity of mind and body), your breath becomes so refined that it is imperceptible. You appear to hold your breath. In fact, your breath has not stopped; it is in suspension, neither breathing nor not breathing.

In this state, your subtle body absorbs the most refined aspect of prana and opens the subtlest conduits of pranic energy, such as *sushumna nadi* (an energy tube running through your spinal canal), through which *kundalini* (special pranic energy in your body) can flow freely. When prana becomes refined, breath becomes sublime, blissful, and spiritually enriching. Then you are breathing the breath of God, the holy breath.

When you learn to control the tiny currents of prana working in your mind, the secret of controlling universal prana is also unlocked. Once this secret is revealed, you fear no power, because you have mastered all the powers in the universe.

Transferring Prana by Osmosis

Pranic energy can be transferred. Anyone coming into proximity with a prana-filled individual receives this energy automatically. The greatest celebrities, the most acclaimed speakers, the most powerful politicians, the most revered prophets, the most successful businesspeople, the most captivating movie stars, the most alluring women—all owe their fame to abundant pranic energy. Magnetic personalities have a knack for influencing others by their speech, even their mere presence.

What is commonly called the "power of persuasion" is simply the capacity to wield pranic energy. Often the most successful, influential, and fascinating people use their pranic power innately, with no conscious knowledge.

Have you ever met someone with a magnetic personality? Were you delighted when you saw him/her, and you loved being near him/her? Did you feel you were basking in his/her energy and vibrations of warmth? Was it hard to tear yourself away? If so, you have experienced the pranic power of charisma.

You may notice similar sensations with someone you love, for pranic energy is shared through kissing and lovemaking. You may be thrilled from head to toe with the electricity of prana, as you exchange energies.

However, the greatest pranic energy is transferred in the presence of spiritual masters. This energy is represented by the halo, portrayed as early as prehistoric cave paintings. Christian paintings and sculptures show a halo around the head of Jesus, the apostles, saints, angels, and religious leaders. Similarly, halos radiate from statues and paintings of Buddha and other deities of the Far East. The Kabbalah, the Jewish mystical teachings written about 500 BC, calls these energies the "astral light."

Have you ever met a spiritual master, saint, or revered person overflowing with pranic energy? Meeting such a living legend is an experience you will never forget. The vast energy radiating from such a being can open you to higher awareness. You may enjoy energy flowing through your body, ecstatic feelings of joy, heady sensations, orgasmic oneness and wholeness, heightened sensory awareness, or waves of love, bliss, and grace.

In India, it is known that holy men and women transmit pranic energy by osmosis. This cosmic energy flow is called *darshan,* a Sanskrit word meaning "sight." So the sight of a saintly person bestows this blessing. Another term for this is *shaktipat,* meaning "transference of *shakti* (pranic energy)." Prana is key to the secret of divine transmission from teacher to student.

For seven years I served on the personal staff of Maharishi Mahesh Yogi, founder of Transcendental Meditation and guru of the Beatles and of Deepak Chopra. On a daily basis I soaked up pranic energy flowing from Maharishi to his disciples. In fact, at that time, I lived for the sublime experience of waves of bliss, joy, and grace that poured from him continually. When he looked into my eyes, I was zapped with pranic energy. My mind expanded, my body vibrated, and my energy field lifted. The closer I got to his energy field, the more pranic energy I felt. That is why his disciples always tried to talk to him, get near him, enter his meeting room, or sit close to him.

The Healing Power of Prana

The founder of Christian Science, Rev. Mary Baker G. Eddy (1821–1910), indicated in her book *Science and Health* that a healing practitioner might reach a state in which the mere presence of the healer is sufficient to effect a successful healing. In this case, all the procedures of affirmations and denials, essential to Christian Science healing, are no longer required. Such was the healing power of Phineas Parkhurst Quimby (1802–1866), an uncanny healer who was Eddy's primary mentor.

The Biblical accounts of Jesus healing, lifting, and inspiring lepers and other diseased people are well known. One woman, hemorrhaging internally for 12 years, spent all her money on physicians, to no avail. As Jesus walked through a crowd, she touched the hem of his cloak. Her bleeding suddenly stopped and she was instantaneously cured. "Somebody hath touched me," Jesus said, "for I perceive that virtue is gone out of me."[4] In another instance, a large group gathered on a plain, asking Jesus for healing: "And the whole multitude sought to touch him: for there went virtue out of him, and healed them all."[5]

"Virtue" is the Biblical name for pranic substance that can be transmitted by a powerful healer of unusual vigor and divine presence. The Latin root of the word virtue is *virtus*, meaning strength, energy, or force, which proceeds from *vir*, the spiritually developed individual, in contrast to mundane emanations from *homo*, the ordinary individual.

This method of pranic healing is referred to in the book of Acts: "Insomuch that they brought forth the sick into the streets, and laid them on beds and couches, that at the least the shadow of Peter passing by might overshadow some of them."[6] This "shadow" is Peter's powerful aura, which healed others by his mere presence through pranic transference. This "contagious health" or "infectious virtue" has been practiced by the yogis of India for eons.

Have you ever stroked a sick friend's forehead or hugged someone in despair? In these loving acts, you are transmitting prana. You can use prana to heal people in need, as long as you know how to replenish it from the infinite source. By consciously increasing prana in your energy field, you can tap vast power resources for self-healing, healing others, even the entire planet.

Never imagine that giving to others will drain you, for the more you impart pranic energy, the more prana flows through you from the cosmic, infinite source. Pranic healing can occur either in person or at a distance via thought transference. Pranic energy can pass through space like a wireless mobile connection.

You can increase your own pranic energy to such a degree that you overcome all obstacles, fulfill all desires, and heal all dis-ease. Any person who truly masters prana conquers not only his own life, but also triumphs over the entire universe.

Sensing Pranic Currents

Pranic energy is undetectable with scientific measurements. Yet, the subtler, more elusive, and more abstract this energy is, the more potent it is. This pranic substance flows through your subtle body in pranic currents. Here I will cover a brief introduction to the basic structure of subtle pranic anatomy. To study this in great depth, please refer to my book *The Power of Chakras*.

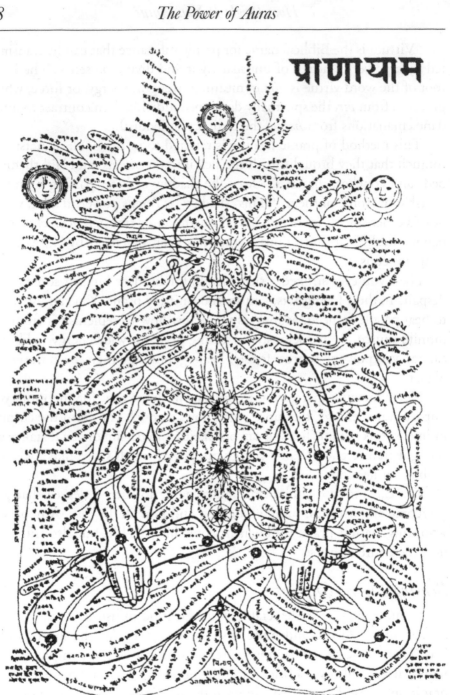

Figure 2a. Nadis

Nadis: Conduits of Subtle Energy

Prana flows through a layer of your subtle body known as the *pranic body*, in fixed pathways called *nadis* ("conduits" or "channels"). According to ancient scriptures of India, there are 72,000 nadis in your pranic body. Some of these nadis are known in China as acupuncture meridians. Your pranic body contains hundreds of centers of concentrated vital energy where many nadis intersect, called *chakras* ("wheels"). Some of these are known as acupuncture points. However, the nadis and chakras are by no means physical. If you dissected a corpse, you would detect no nadi or chakra anywhere.

The three most important nadis through which prana flows are called *sushumna, ida,* and *pingala*. Sushumna is the median channel reaching from the base of your spine, near the tailbone, all the way up through the top of your skull. The caduceus, symbol of the American Medical Association, is a depiction of ida and pingala coiling around this central canal. Although most doctors have no knowledge of nadis, the ida and pingala govern the parasympathetic and sympathetic aspects of your autonomic nervous system, respectively. Sushumna nadi is the conduit of *kundalini,* often called "serpent power" or "mystic coil"—a special cosmic pranic energy that remains dormant until it is awakened, usually through spiritual practices.

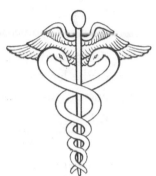

Figure 2b. Caduceus

The term *kundalini* derives from the Sanskrit root *kundal* ("curled up"), because in ordinary humans, it remains dormant, coiled at the base of the spine. As kundalini wakes up and rises up the spine, it opens the chakras, bringing health, well-being, energy, and, ultimately, spiritual enlightenment.

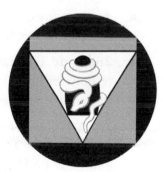

Figure 2c. Kundalini

Your 10 major nadis are connected to 10 "gates"—orifices of the body through which the vital life-force or prana may exit the body at death. These are called *manovahi nadis,* or *yoga nadis,* through which pranic currents operate the sympathetic and parasympathetic nervous systems. When kundalini awakens, all of these nadis are activated:

- ⚕ **10th gate** (fontanel at crown): *Sushumna nadi* begins at the base of the spine and extends up through the top of the skull. This is the nadi through which kundalini passes.

- ⚕ **9th gate** (left nostril): *Ida nadi,* the lunar or female nadi, begins at the base of the spine and extends to the left nostril. It conserves energy and calms the mind.

- ⚕ **8th gate** (right nostril): *Pingala nadi,* the solar or male nadi, begins at the base of the spine and extends to the right nostril. It provides physical strength, endurance, and speed.

- ⚕ **7th gate** (left eye): *Gandhari nadi* extends from the big toe of the left foot to the corner of the left eye. It carries subtle energy from the lower body to the third eye chakra.

- ⚕ **6th gate** (right eye): *Hastajihva nadi* extends from the big toe of the left foot to the corner of the right eye.

- ⚕ **5th gate** (left ear): *Yashasvini nadi* extends from the right big toe to the left ear.

- ⚕ **4th gate** (right ear): *Pusha nadi* extends from the left big toe to the right ear.

- ⚕ **3rd gate** (mouth): *Alambusha nadi,* associated with assimilation and elimination, begins at the anus and terminates in the mouth.

- ⚕ **2nd gate** (genitals): *Kuhu nadi* begins at the throat and terminates in the genitals. It carries the subtle energy, *bindu,* responsible for ejaculation.

- ⚕ **1st gate** (anus): *Shankhini nadi* begins in the throat and extends to the anus. It is activated in the practice of enemas and other purificatory practices.

Most animals leave the body through the first or second gates. They defecate or urinate at death. Humans usually leave through the third to ninth gates—the open mouth or eyes, or bleeding eyes or nose. Only yogis leave the body through the 10th gate at the crown—the gate through which spiritual liberation is attained. This gate is open at birth as a soft spot but closes after six months. Read my books *The Power of Chakras* and *Exploring Meditation* to learn practices that can reopen that gate.

Subtle Energy Centers

To write my award-winning book *Exploring Chakras*, later released as *The Power of Chakras*, I researched the Vedic and Tantric scriptures of ancient India to find the most authentic information about the subject. In that book I cover the 14 main chakras mentioned in the scriptures: seven major chakras that you may already be familiar with, and seven others that you might not be aware of. Many of these are in your skull or above your head.

Let us first learn to pronounce the word *chakra*. I know this may be challenging, considering that you are reading this book rather than hearing it. But right now, say the name Chuck. Now say the word run. Now put the two together, but eliminate the "n" at the end of the word run, and replace it with an "h."

"Chuck-ruh."

That is (approximately) how to say the word chakra. There is no such pronunciation as "shock-rah" in the Sanskrit language or in the English language. "Shock-rah" is how most people mispronounce the word. I am currently on a worldwide campaign to teach everyone how to pronounce the word chakra correctly: "chuck-ruh."

Chakra is a Sanskrit word meaning "wheel." Why is it a wheel? Because it has a hub and spokes. The hub is where many conduits of pranic energy intersect, and the spokes are radiations of pranic energy. So a chakra is a concentrated center of pranic energy in the layer of your subtle body known as your pranic body.

The 14 main chakras through which kundalini energy flows are as follows:

1. *Muladhara: Mula* means "base" or "root," because it is at the base of your spine near the tailbone. It is responsible for excretion, sense of smell, and earth element, and it is associated with the adrenal glands.

Location of Major Chakra Points

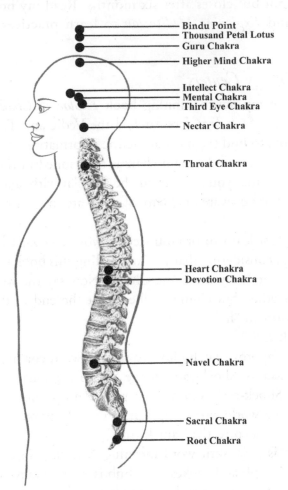

Bindu Point
Thousand Petal Lotus
Guru Chakra
Higher Mind Chakra

Intellect Chakra
Mental Chakra
Third Eye Chakra

Nectar Chakra

Throat Chakra

Heart Chakra
Devotion Chakra

Navel Chakra

Sacral Chakra
Root Chakra

Figure 2d.

2. *Svadhishthana* means "one's own self," because it is where individuality comes into embodiment through procreation. The second chakra, in the sacral region, governs sexuality, reproduction, sense of taste, and water element. It is associated with the gonads.

Chakra Points in Brain

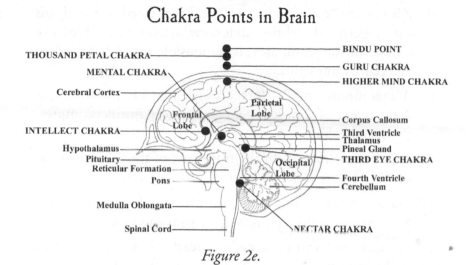

Figure 2e.

3. *Manipura* means "city of jewels," where 101 conduits of pranic energy intersect and where the fires of digestion burn. The navel chakra, in the lumbar region, oversees digestion, sense of sight, and fire element. It is associated with the pancreas.

4. *Anahata* means "unstruck sound," because the unstruck sound is the sound of silence—where divine consciousness resides. The heart chakra, in the thoracic region, is the seat of your soul, the gateway to higher consciousness. It manages the sense of touch and air element, and it is associated with the thymus gland.

5. *Hrit* means "heart." Right below the anahata chakra, it is the seat of devotion to God and of fulfillment of all desires.

6. *Vishuddha* means "purification." The throat chakra, in the cervical region, deals with sense of hearing, ether element, and creative expression. It is associated with the thyroid gland.

7. *Talu,* the nectar chakra, in the medulla oblongata, is related to the uvula, the flow of *soma* (nectar of immortality), and the current of pranic energy.

8. *Ajna* means "command center" and is situated in the glands that regulate the entire endocrine system. The third eye chakra, in the pineal area, is responsible for higher wisdom and clairvoyant sight.

9. *Manas* means "mind." In the upper part of ajna chakra, it is the center of your lower mental vehicle: instincts, impressions, and habits.

10. *Indu* means "moon." In the front part of the brain, it is the seat of intellect and higher mind.

11. *Nirvana* means "dissolution." At the top of your brain, it is associated with the annihilation of your ego.

12. *Guru* means "light/darkness" or "teacher." Above your head in the lower part of sahasrara chakra, it is the center in which divine light dispels the darkness of ignorance.

13. *Sahasrara* means "thousandfold." The thousand-petaled lotus above your head, it is the center of divine union, integration, enlightenment, and illumination.

14. *Bindu* means "point." In the upper sahasrara chakra, it is the center of infinitely concentrated energy, the fountainhead from which your entire energy system springs.

Figure 2f on page 45 illustrates how the chakras form a Star of David. The upper triangle represents cosmic life, and the lower triangle symbolizes earthly life, which, when integrated, bring higher consciousness. Figure 2g on page 45 expands that star into a three-dimensional star tetrahedron, often called the *merkabah*. The true form of this star is the Kabbalistic Tree of Life pattern in Figure 2h. (See page 46 for this illustration.)

Chakra Correlations

Your seven major chakras are associated with specific colors, planets, days of the week, and gemstones. These correlations are found in the scriptures of ancient India. You might think you already know what colors correspond to various chakras. However, the true, esoteric colors are

Star of David: Heaven on Earth

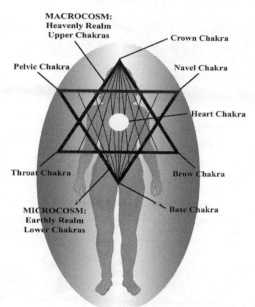

Figure 2f.

Star Tetrahedron

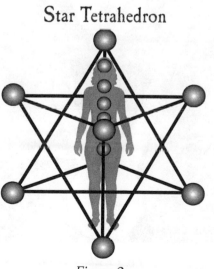

Figure 2g.

Tree of Life

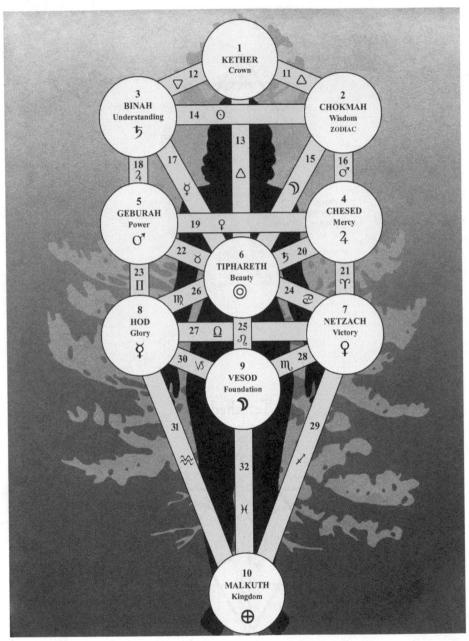

Figure 2h.

something quite different. Therefore the teaching in this section will not correspond with conventional ideas. These colors and planets are based on ancient Vedic astrology, called *Jyotish*.

The days of the week form a rainbow that begins on Sunday. Therefore, Sunday is red, Monday is orange, Tuesday is yellow, Wednesday is green, Thursday is blue, Friday is indigo, and Saturday is violet:

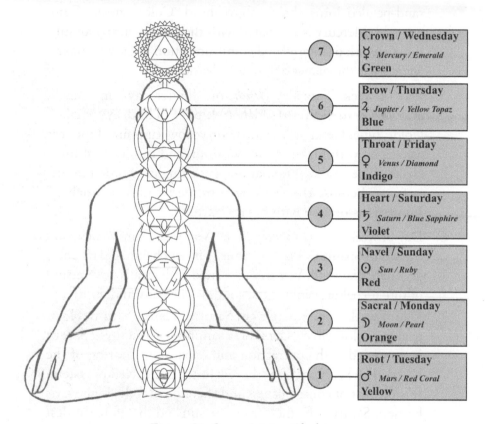

Figure 2i. Seven Major Chakras

1. Day of week: Sunday (Day of the Sun). Planet: Sun. Solar (Sun) plexus chakra. Color: red. Gem: ruby. The Sun is associated with vital energy and the fire of digestion of navel chakra.

2. Day of week: Monday (Day of the Moon). Planet: Moon. Sacral chakra. Color: orange. Gem: pearl or moonstone. The Moon is associated with emotions, fecundity, and fertility of sacral chakra.

3. Day of week: Tuesday (*Mardi,* or "Mars day," in French, and *Martes* in Spanish). Planet: Mars. Root chakra. Color: yellow. Gem: red coral. Mars is associated with primal needs and survival instincts of root chakra. Mars is the God of war.

4. Day of week: Wednesday (*Mercredi,* or "Mercury day," in French, and *Miércoles* in Spanish). Planet: Mercury. Thousand-petaled lotus chakra above head. Color: green. Gem: emerald. Mercury is associated with the brain—nearly an infinite network of interrelated communication in crown chakra. Mercury is the planet of communication.

5. Day of week: Thursday (*Jeudi,* or "Jupiter day," in French, and *Jueves* in Spanish). Planet: Jupiter. Third eye chakra. Color: blue. Gem: yellow topaz or yellow sapphire. Jupiter is associated with higher mind, wisdom, and intuition of brow chakra. The Sanskrit translation of the English word "Jupiter" is *Guru.* Because the word *guru* primarily means "teacher," Jupiter is associated with higher learning.

6. Day of week: Friday *(Vendredi,* or "Venus day," in French, and *Viernes* in Spanish). Planet: Venus. Throat chakra. Color: indigo. Gem: diamond. Venus is associated with creative expression of throat chakra. Venus is the goddess of beauty and creativity.

7. Day of week: Saturday (Day of Saturn). Planet: Saturn. Heart chakra. Color: violet. Gem: blue sapphire or amethyst. Saturn is associated with contraction and expansion (beating of the heart). The heart chakra is the key to the entire chakra system. It is the seat of consciousness and therefore has the highest vibration. Saturn is furthest from the sun and therefore subtlest and highest of the seven inner planets.

You can learn much more about your subtle energy system, chakras, kundalini, and pranic energy by reading *The Power of Chakras,* where you will find profound information not found in any other book.

In the next chapter, you will explore the amazing, multidimensional world of your subtle body, which comprises your auric field.

3

Your Multifaceted Aura

ಸಂ

Exploring Subtle Body Anatomy

"Departing this world [one] attains this Annamaya self, this Pranamaya self does he attain, this Manomaya self he attains, this Vijnanamaya self he attains, he attains this Anandamaya self."

—The Upanishads[1]

Have you ever dreamt you were falling, and then you suddenly woke up with a jolt? Have you dreamt you were flying above the rooftops as Superman does? Have you ever catapulted out of your body and then, when you looked down at your body, thought it belonged to someone else?

If these descriptions sound familiar, then you have experienced your subtle body firsthand. Often your subtle body temporarily separates from your physical body during sleep. It may hover over your body or even fly above your home. If your subtle body suddenly drops back into your physical body, you might wake with a shock or shudder when the two bodies reunite.

What do I mean by *subtle body*? You are well aware that you have a gross physical body, which requires food, sleep, and exercise. However, you also have a subtle body, made of light, thought, and pranic energy. Your subtle body needs different nourishment than your physical body. When fed spiritual food, such as prayer, meditation, and positive thinking, it

49

becomes robust and healthy. When fed negative thoughts and toxic emotions, it shrinks and collapses.

In this chapter you will discover and explore the multifaceted layers and dimensions of this human energy field.

Your Energy Body

Nearly every civilization gives credence to an animating spirit, invisible essence, electric force field, aura, or luminous subtle body that pervades and encompasses the physical body. This spiritual body is visible only to subtle sense perception—clairvoyance, clairaudience, and clairsentience. This light-body can dissociate from your physical body during sleep, hypnosis, meditation, or near-death experiences, or under anesthesia. At death it permanently splits from your gross body, yet continues to live in higher realms of existence.

Because your energy body is larger than your physical body, it extends past your gross body's boundaries, and its outer edge is visible as an aura. This light-body may appear multilayered, egg-shaped, spiral, or oval, or it may follow the body's contours. It seems thicker or denser close to the body, and more vaporous and transparent at its outer edges. Yet, the aura's influence is felt farther away than even the best clairvoyant sight can perceive.

This energy body has many names: aura, auric field, subtle body, astral body, etheric body, etheric double, doppelganger, fluidic body, Beta body, counterpart body, pre-physical body, bioplasmic body, psychic atmosphere, or magnetic atmosphere.

Phantom Leaves in Labs

High-frequency photography was invented in the early 20th century when Semyon Kirlian, a Russian electrotherapy technician, first photographed the aura in a field of high-frequency electrical currents. Using Kirlian's camera, Soviet scientists extensively studied the luminous body of animate and inanimate objects during the 20th century.

In *Psychic Discoveries Behind the Iron Curtain,* Ostrander and Schroeder first described the "phantom leaf" effect. After cutting off a section of a plant leaf, researchers found a glowing leaf pattern still visible in their photographs, as though the entire leaf still existed in light form.

Scientists conjectured that the leaf's energy field is a holograph that underlies physical matter and may be responsible for organizing its structure. They named this field the *biological plasma body*, or *bioplasma*, which remains even when a part of the organism is cut away. When this light-body disappears, the plant or animal dies.

Though American researchers could not replicate the Soviet experiments, many scientists still believed this discovery was highly significant. Finally, in 1973, after more than 500 trials, Kendall Johnson photographed a phantom leaf with clear internal details. Yet his finding was dismissed as an electrostatic artifact.

John Hubacher, a graduate student in the high-frequency photography laboratory of Thelma Moss at University of California at Los Angeles (UCLA), was more successful. About five percent of his attempts showed the clear, detailed internal structure of the cut-off section of the leaf. Twenty percent resulted in partial images.

Later, in the same UCLA laboratory, Clark Dugger, a graduate student in the UCLA cinema department, took slow-motion pictures of the phantom leaf effect at about six frames per second with both black-and-white and color film through a special transparent electrode. With this method, brilliant phantom leaves shimmered and vibrated for a few seconds and then vanished. Dugger always used springtime leaves that were cut just before being placed on the electrode.[2]

The startling phantom leaf effect may account for experiences of amputees with phantom limbs, who continue to feel pain, aching, tingling, itching, or numbness in a missing arm or leg. Psychologist Ron Melzack of McGill University in Montreal studied 125 people with missing limbs, mostly teenagers. He concluded, "In fact, you do not need the body to feel the body."[3] Physicians typically view this as a wishful-thinking hallucination to view the body as it once was. But clairvoyants claim to actually see phantom limbs—the missing arm or leg in subtle form, still attached to the body.

You Are Light and Sound

During thousands of typical near-death experiences (NDEs), survivors report seeing subtle light-bodies clearly. When Dannion Brinkley, author of *Saved by the Light*, was struck by lightning, he catapulted out of his body where, in his light body, he viewed the proceedings from high above

Roadmap of Your Auric Field

Body	Sheath	Faculties	Level of Identity	Motives
Gross Body	Food Sheath	1. Earth 4. Air 2. Water 5. Ether 3. Fire	Environment	1. Projection 4. Control 2. Creativity 5. Competition 3. Movement 6. Relationship
Gross Body	Food Sheath	1. 5 Sense Organs 2. 5 Organs of Action 3. 5 Elements	Physical Body	1. Birth 4. Change 2. Survival 5. Decay 3. Growth 6. Death
Gross Body	Vital Sheath	1. 5 Vital Airs 2. 5 Subtle Elements 3. 5 Working Senses	Instinctual Mind	1. Desire 4. Sleep 2. Action 5. Fear 3. Propagation 6. Appetite
Subtle Body	Mental Sheath	1. Thinking 3. Deliberation 2. Perception 4. Experience	Conscious Mind	1. Attention 3. Reasoning 2. Selection 4. Perception
Subtle Body	Mental Sheath	1. Memories 4. Sensations 2. Impressions 5. Feelings 3. 5 Knowing Senses	Subconscious Sensory Mind	1. Sensory Experiences 2. Storing Impressions 3. Storing Memories
Subtle Body	Mental Sheath	1. Habits 4. Patterns 2. Conditions 5. Beliefs 3. Aptitudes 6. Talents	Subconscious Habit Mind	1. Defense 3. Emotion 2. Reaction 4. Fluctuation 3. Retaining 5. Habituation
Subtle Body	Intellect Sheath	1. Cognition 3. Knowledge 2. Intelligence 4. Discriminaton	Intellect	1. Discernment 3. Generalizing 2. Decision 4. Understanding
Subtle Body	Intellect Sheath	1. Separation 3. Acceptance 2. Identity 4. Rejection	Ego	1. Will 3. Power 2. Demand 4. Security

Façade Barrier (False Belief in Separation from God)

	Sheath	Level of Identity	Faculties	Motives
Causal Body	**Blissful Sheath**	**Higher Mind Etheric Soul Self**	1. Clairvoyance 2. Clairsentience 3. Clairaudience 4. Immortality 5. Intuition	1. True Desires, Purpose 2. True Identity, Expression 3. Freedom of Choice 4. Continuity, Purity
Higher Bodies		**Christ Self**	1. Christ Love 2. Christ Light 3. Teaching 4. Salvation 5. Joy, Peace 6. Lifting 7. Comfort 8. Protection	1. Inner Guidance, Comforting 2. Blessing, Healing, Protecting 3. Forgiving, Redeeming 4. Unconditional Love
	Spiritual Sheaths	**"I AM" Self**	1. Existence 2. Awareness 3. Beingness 4. Serenity 5. Wisdom, Truth 6. Knowingness 7. Teaching 8. Fulfillment	1. Strength, Authority, Dominion 2. Realizing "I AM That I AM" 3. Expressing Divine Destiny 4. Inner Truth, Self-Realization
		God Self	1. God-Presence 2. God-Power 3. Divine Light 4. Divine Love 5. Glory, Grace 6. Oneness 7. Wholeness 8. Holiness	1. Sanctification 2. Unification with God 3. Devotion and Surrender 4. Divine Love and Light
		Cosmic Self	1. Universe 2. Cosmos 3. Galactic 4. Vastness 5. All Creation 6. All Time 7. All Space 8. Enormity	1. Expansion, Permanence 2. All-Pervasiveness 3. Embodying the Cosmos 4. Universality, Eternity
Present Everywhere		**Absolute Pure Consciousness**	1. Formless 2. Nameless 3. Infinity 4. Indivisibility 5. Attributeless 6. Omnipotence 7. Omniscience 8. Transcendent	1. Perfection Everywhere Now 2. Contentment, Balance, Harmony 3. Radiance, Peace, Enlightenment 4. Uninvolved Witness of Creation

Figure 3a.

his physical form. From this vantage point he perceived loved ones scurrying about, trying to save his life. Yet Dannion saw more than just their physical, material bodies. They were filled with multicolored radiant light. However, Dannion's physical body, lying lifeless on the floor, was stonelike, with no luminosity. Then Dannion, who was floating up near the ceiling in his light body, looked at his own arm, hand, and fingers. Surprisingly, they were shimmering with brilliant effulgence.[4]

Everyone is a multidimensional being of light, living in a universe of luminous spheres. This statement may sound fantastic, yet it concurs with modern physics. Superstring theory envisions a 10- or 11-dimensional space-time. And the elementary particles observed in particle accelerators are nothing more than excitation modes of elementary strings—vibrating waves of energy.

Just like everything else in creation, you are a bundle of pulsating, shimmering bodies of light and sound. Your stream of consciousness reaches from the divine level through all subtle levels to your gross physical body. You have a separate identity on each level, and you live on all levels simultaneously. Myriad inner identities comprise your one identity, and many subtle vibrational bodies make up your inner form.

It is said in the Bible, "There are also celestial bodies, and bodies terrestrial."[5] and "There is a natural body, and there is a spiritual body."[6] Ernest Holmes, founder of the Church of Religious Science, states, "It is our belief that we do have a body within a body to infinity."[7]

Your physical shell, which you temporarily inhabit, is just one of your many multilayered, multidimensional bodies. Subtle bodies of pure liquid light, in myriad brilliant crystalline hues, pervade your physical frame and extend beyond it.

Your bodies vibrate at specific frequencies. The vibratory rate of dense physical matter is slower than light, which has the highest frequency. Thus, your physical body vibrates at a slower pace than subtle bodies. Your subtlest body vibrates at the highest frequency. Grosser bodies are more individualized. Subtler, more abstract levels of identity are more universal. Bodies on higher frequencies are less subject to laws of time and space than bodies of denser vibration.

A clairvoyant may see light-bodies inside, above, beside, or near your physical frame. On the highest vibrational levels, your indwelling Spirit lives in several bodies concurrently. Subtle bodies are not necessarily confined to your gross body's boundaries. Inner bodies may exist in several places simultaneously, for there is no time or space in Spirit.

As you explore your energy field, you will realize what a powerful, radiant light-being you are. You will uncover dimensional realities beyond imagination. The amazing world of your own luminous sphere will open as you discover multifarious components of your aura being.

Now let us explore the outer and inner bodies that comprise your energy field. (See Figure 3a on pages 52 and 53.)

Your Cosmic Anatomy

Your many levels of awareness embody corresponding auric layers. Within your radiant body of light, various parts of your subtle body vibrate at unique, discrete frequencies. The yogis of ancient India say that you have a threefold body: gross physical body, subtle body, and causal or seed body. Within these three bodies are several sheaths: physical, vital, mental, intellect, and blissful sheaths. Your subtler bodies and sheaths surround and permeate the grosser ones in multidimensional layers.

The layers of your auric field are detailed extensively in my books *Exploring Meditation* and *The Power of Chakras.* Information about the layers of your higher self are covered in *Divine Revelation.* Please refer to these books for further study. Here, you will learn some additional information not covered in these previous books.

Your Gross Physical Body

Your gross physical body is called the *food sheath* because it is made of food, requires food, dies without food, and, after death, becomes food for insects. Like a mechanical robot, this fragile, perishable, temporary vehicle performs actions as though it were alive, yet it has no will or life of its own. It is entirely controlled by your mind.

Made of five elements, your food sheath is solid due to earth element, fluid due to water, warm due to fire, active and moving due to air, and occupying space due to ether.

Your food sheath was originally designed to manifest a perfect form: symmetrical, youthful, and beautiful. However, it is distorted by erroneous beliefs, including limitation, illness, aging, and death. Thus, your mental body is the construct upon which your food sheath is built.

Sheaths of the Human Energy Field

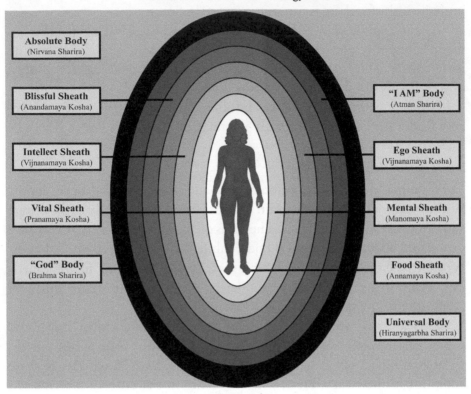

Absolute Body
(Nirvana Sharira)

Blissful Sheath
(Anandamaya Kosha)

Intellect Sheath
(Vijnanamaya Kosha)

Vital Sheath
(Pranamaya Kosha)

"God" Body
(Brahma Sharira)

"I AM" Body
(Atman Sharira)

Ego Sheath
(Vijnanamaya Kosha)

Mental Sheath
(Manomaya Kosha)

Food Sheath
(Annamaya Kosha)

Universal Body
(Hiranyagarbha Sharira)

Figure 3b.

Your Subtle Body

Your subtle body consists of three sheaths: vital, mental, and intellect sheaths, made of 18 principles: intellect, ego, mind, five knowing senses, five working senses, and five sense objects. These generate the five elements of your gross physical body. Sound produces the element of ether, touch gives rise to air, form to fire, flavor to water, and odor to earth. Here is a brief summary of the components of the five elements:

1. Ether is the vehicle for sound: 100-percent sound.

2. Air is the vehicle for touch: 50-percent sound and 50-percent touch.

3. Fire is the vehicle for form: 33.3-percent sound, 33.3-percent touch, and 33.3-percent form.

Elements of Gross and Subtle Bodies

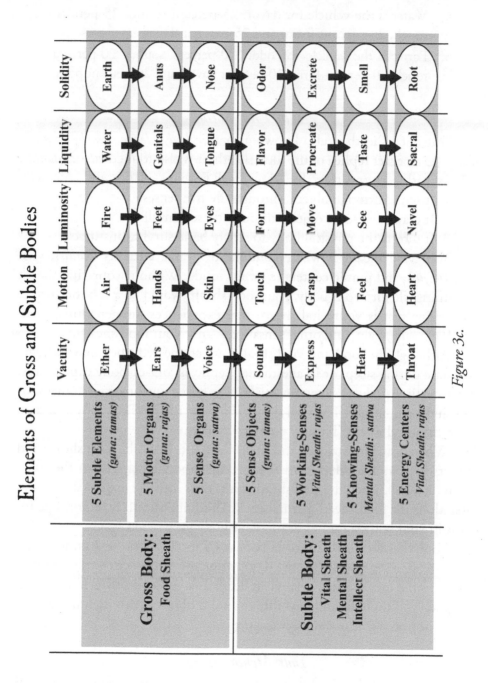

Figure 3c.

4. Water is the vehicle for flavor: 25-percent sound, 25-percent touch, 25-percent form, and 25-percent flavor.
5. Earth is the vehicle for odor: 20-percent sound, 20-percent touch, 20-percent form, 20-percent flavor, and 20-percent odor.

Your Vital Sheath

Your vital sheath is also known as *pranic body*, *desire sheath*, or *astral body*. As an exact replica of the food sheath, it is also termed *etheric double*. This sheath performs three functions in all humans, plants, and animals:

1. It senses external objects through the five senses.
2. It craves the sense objects through these stimuli.
3. It directs the physical body to satisfy basic survival instincts.

Your vital sheath is where conduits of pranic currents (*nadis*), vital airs (*vayus*), and pranic centers (*chakras*) reside. Without your vital sheath breathing life into your body, your food sheath would be a robotic corpse. Surprisingly, it is your vital sheath that experiences hunger, thirst, heat, cold, pleasure, pain, and other sensations—not your food sheath.

Although the food and vital sheaths are connected, they may partially separate during sleep, or in anesthesia, hypnosis, out-of-body experiences, near-death experiences, certain meditative states, unconscious trances, or psychic mediumship. The vital sheath can leave the physical body and travel in the astral world. This is called *astral travel*.

When death approaches, the vital sheath lifts from the food sheath and hovers over it. The silver cord that attaches the vital sheath to the navel snaps at death. Then the vital sheath withdraws into the mental sheath and abandons the food sheath permanently. Your vital sheath is responsible for heat in your body. Thus, at death, your body grows cold.

Your vital sheath is said to pulsate at 15 to 20 cycles per minute. Aura readers often see it as light blue to gray lines of force from one-quarter of an inch to 2 inches wide. It survives death as a ghost or spirit. It can travel as quickly as thought and pass through solid objects. Although it may feel dense or heavy, it is not subject to gravity.

Your Mental Sheath

Your mental sheath, the second aspect of your subtle body, consists of three parts: conscious or lower mind, subconscious sensory mind, and reflexive mind. All aspects of your mental sheath cooperate to produce your every experience.

- ⚜ **Conscious Mind.** Your conscious mind performs mental functions and directs actions. It has the capacity to think, deliberate, and reason. Your mental body is built of thought-forms and ideas projected from your mind. It is clear and vibrant in highly evolved people and often displays fine energy lines of bright yellow light. This mental body often follows the outline of your physical body and extends 3 to 6 inches beyond its boundaries. This glow is more pronounced around the head, forming a halo.

- ⚜ **Subconscious Sensory Mind.** Whereas your conscious mind is the objective, active mind, your subconscious sensory-impression mind is subjective and passive. Your subconscious body, also known as emotional body, links your soul with your conscious mind. This body can project from your physical body and travel at the speed of thought. Without heaviness or mass, it occupies no space and is not subject to gravity. It continues after death. This auric layer vibrates with myriad deep, intense colors, changing according to moods. Dominating colors indicate which emotions are prevalent. Composed of dense rainbow clouds in continual, fluid motion, this emotional body extends 3 to 6 inches beyond the physical body's boundaries.

- ⚜ **Subconscious Habit Mind (Reflexive Mind).** Your reflexive, patterned mind consists of subliminal traits, inclinations, and habits that create repetitive expectations and complex, emotionally charged reactions. Your subconscious habit-mind body is also called *index body*, because it tabulates experiences. Your subconscious habit body is part of your emotional body, described previously.

Your Intellect Sheath

The intellect sheath is the third aspect of your subtle body. It functions as a semi-permanent vehicle, created millions of years ago, when you first passed from animal incarnation into human form. Its two components are intellect and ego. Your intellect is your seat of cognition, intelligence, intuition, and knowledge, which can decide, resolve, generalize, retain, and understand abstract ideas. Your ego is your individual human identity. Considering itself a separate entity, it mistakes itself to be your true self.

Refer again to Figure 3a on page 52 and 53. The façade barrier, or psychic barrier, is an illusory mental wall dividing your ego from your real self. This illusion of duality is a façade or mask. The true, loving self of harmony and God-like qualities is hidden by this false ego.

Your intellect/ego sheath, also known as the *connector body*, bridges your lower self to your higher self. Aura readers see it as amorphous rainbow clouds of color, light in density, about 6 to 12 inches beyond the body. It is sometimes infused with the color rose.

What Happens to Subtle Body After Death?

Your subtle body does not change at death. Your higher self, clothed in your subtle body, abandons your physical body and moves to higher dimensions, accompanied by your mind, prana, senses, and all other subtle elements—the seeds of your new body.

Once your higher self flees your body, the chief prana departs. Then all other pranas follow. (See my book *The Power of Chakras* for a detailed description of pranas.) The pranas cannot remain in the body without the subtle elements and subtle organs, which form the bedrock on which pranas flow. Your soul cannot enter a new body without prana.

Your capacities and tendencies endure after death. They determine your afterlife and mold future incarnations. Everything you ever experienced is stored in your subconscious memory bank. When you are reborn, you wear the same subtle body that has persisted throughout all cycles of incarnation.

Your Causal Body

Your causal body is the seed of ignorance, because it causes both gross and subtle bodies to exist by virtue of the false ego, from which all experiences arise.

Blissful Sheath

Only one sheath comprises your causal body: blissful sheath, which emits the blissfulness of the higher self, yet covers the higher self like a sheath. This body is but a shadow of the true higher self—the *atman*, or "I AM," self.

Your causal body, also known as *etheric-soul-self body*, forms your unique individuality, expressing your heart's desires and soul's purpose for this incarnation. Although your physical body changes, the soul body is ever-youthful, flawless, vibrant, luminous, beautiful, and effervescent, with perfect symmetry and divine radiance. This body assumes the same sex as your physical body during any given incarnation.

Your blissful sheath (etheric template or etheric soul-self body) is the higher, perfect template of your physical body, which wears the mental, astral, and physical bodies as distorted masks covering its true glory.

This effulgent blissful sheath displays beautiful pastel colors radiating light. It can appear in a form that resembles the physical body. To many aura readers it looks like a photographic negative of your physical

body, extending 12 to 24 inches beyond the body. However, I have measured it extending 10 feet or more beyond the physical body's boundaries in healthy, spiritual individuals.

Higher Bodies

Beyond your fivefold sheath are your higher bodies, which can dwell in many places at once, working with many different people on universal and personal levels simultaneously.

"Christ" Body

Here the name "Christ" is not synonymous solely with Jesus. It is a universal level of

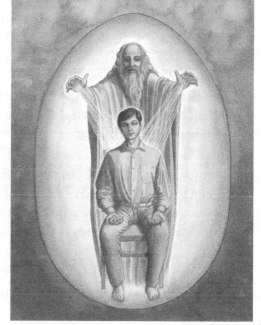

Figure 3d. Your Higher Self

consciousness not bound by particular religious traditions, a level of inner identity within people of all backgrounds. The word *Christ* comes from the Greek word *christos*, meaning "the anointed." Thus, your Christ-self is your inner Christ, the "anointed one" living in Spirit within you. It is your higher self, the Christ Consciousness, which expresses the most ideal qualities of human life.

Your Christ-self body may appear with various forms and names, which specialize in areas of life that you are working on at the time. Christ-selves may be male or female, depending on which is more appropriate for a particular area of learning.

Your Christ-self may hover above your head as a divine protector, guardian angel, celestial being, or globe of light. However, it is part of your higher self, rather than a power outside yourself. Composed of Spirit, it is subject to no physical laws. Some aura readers see this celestial body as beautiful shimmering lines of rainbow light, extending from 24 to 36 inches beyond the physical body.

"I AM" Body

Your higher self is called *atman*, the mighty "I AM" presence. Your "I AM," or "I exist," is the most abstract, fundamental, universal component of your individuality. The individuation of the impersonal God, whereby universal consciousness manifests as individual consciousness in order to communicate or express, the "I AM" self is universal wisdom, love, and truth made manifest. The purpose of the "I AM" is to fulfill God's purpose through you as an individual.

Your "I AM" self lives in the "I AM" body. It usually appears in both male and female form and has two names, one male and one female. To some aura readers, the "I AM"–self body (spiritual sheath, or *ketheric body*) appears as tiny gold and silver threads of light forming a grid-like structure supporting your human body.

God Body

Your God-self is your direct connection to the almighty personal God of your understanding, in whatever form you believe that to be. The purpose of your God-self is to unify individual consciousness with God consciousness. Your God-self is the personal form of God realized as your higher self.

Your God-self may be any beloved deity, whether Krishna, Durga, Jesus, Mother Mary, Buddha, Jehovah, Hashem, Allah, or another form. The

God-self is universal, without characteristics associated with you as an individual. However you can own these characteristics as a God-realized being.

The embodiment of the God-self is the divine body of the personal God. You probably have one male and one female God-self name and form. Aura readers might perceive the God-self as a face or form of God or sphere of divine light and unconditional love above you.

Cosmic Body

Your cosmic self is wholly universal in nature. The universal "I AM" presence, it is the omnipresent intelligence of the universe. As vast as the universe, it embodies and encompasses all the stars, galaxies, and space of the cosmos. All life is contained within the cosmic self, and the cosmic self dwells within each individual.

Your cosmic-self body is the cosmos, and its nature is universal consciousness. It is neither male nor female; you probably have one cosmic-self name and one form. The cosmic self works with cosmic life, and its function is universal.

Absolute Body

The absolute body is not a body. It is without form, phenomena, or boundaries. In this bodiless body, everything disappears. Singularity, oneness, and wholeness remain. Here you merge with universal Spirit in supreme enlightenment and absolute truth. You are free from bondage and attain the highest beatitude.

This level of consciousness is pure universal awareness, the silent witness of all creation, pure silence, without thought, activity, or fluctuation. Its inner state, *samadhi* (evenness of mind), can be experienced in deep meditation.

Absolute pure consciousness is beyond other levels of identity and also permeates all levels. The ultimate principle of life, it underlies, upholds, and sustains the universe by its very being. The impersonal aspect of God, beyond time, space, limitation, and causation, it is infinite, nameless, formless, and without personal identity, light, color, marks, or characteristics.

The absolute is your true nature of being—unmanifest, unchanging, eternal, unbounded, and separate from your various bodies and sheaths. Yet you mistakenly identify with these bodies and sheaths, such as ego and

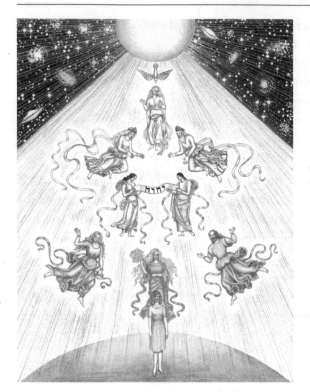

Figure 3e. Your Higher Bodies

intellect. That is not who you are. You are, in essence, a limitless being of pure, immortal consciousness.

Please refer to Figure 3e, which depicts many bodies of your higher self. Just above the woman is her individual, immortal, etheric soul-self (*jiva*), holding a bouquet of roses. Universal aspects of her higher self surround her. Two figures floating above her represent her male and female Christ-selves. The two figures holding a scroll with the Hebrew letters *Yod He Vav He* ("I AM That I AM," or *Yahweh*) are her male and female "I AM" selves (*atman*). The two aspects of her God-self (*ishvara*) are wearing crowns. The female figure just below the dove is the feminine aspect of God, called Holy Spirit. The stars and galaxies represent the cosmic self. The golden sun is the impersonal supreme Godhead (*Brahman*) shining its radiance everywhere, which represents absolute pure consciousness: *satchitananda*.

The Seven Worlds

As a multidimensional being, each of your inner bodies dwells in a separate dimension. This claim may sound unbelievable, but today's theoretical physics postulates that we live in many dimensions simultaneously. The ancient scriptures of India speak of seven cosmic regions corresponding to your seven sheaths and seven major chakras. Of these seven realms, the three highest are called worlds of Brahma.

Multidimensional Auric Field

Bodies	*Sheaths*	*Realms*	*Chakras*
Absolute Body *(Nirvana Sharira)* Brahmin Consciousness	**Unmanifest Self** *(Paramashiva)*	**Beyond All Worlds** *(Paramashiva)*	**Point** *(Bindu)* Oneness
God Body *(Brahma Sharira)* God Consciousness	**Supreme Self** *(Brahma Sthiti)*	**God World** *(Brahma Loka)*	**Crown** *(Sahasrara)* Love
"I AM" Body *(Atman Sharira)* Transcendence	**Higher Self** *(Atma Sthiti)*	**Truth World** *(Satya Loka)*	**Brilliant** *(Guru)* Light
Causal Body *(Karana Sharira)* Deep Sleep State	**Blissful Sheath** *(Anandamaya Kosha)*	**Perfect World** *(Tapah Loka)*	**Brow** *(Ajna)* Mind
	Ego Sheath *(Vijnanamaya Kosha)*	**Subliminal World** *(Janah Loka)*	**Throat** *(Vishuddha)* Ether Element
Subtle Body *(Sukshma Sharira)* Dream State	**Intellect Sheath** *(Vijnanamaya Kosha)*	**Middle World** *(Mahah Loka)*	**Heart** *(Anahata)* Air Element
	Mental Sheath *(Manomaya Kosha)*	**Subtle World** *(Svah Loka)*	**Navel** *(Manipura)* Fire Element
	Vital Sheath *(Pranamaya Kosha)*	**Astral World** *(Bhuvah Loka)*	**Sacral** *(Svadhishthana)* Water Element
Gross Body *(Stula Sharira)* Waking State	**Food Sheath** *(Annamaya Kosha)*	**Physical World** *(Bhu Loka)*	**Root** *(Muladhara)* Earth Element

Figure 3f.

1. Your food sheath dwells in *earth realm*, the material world, earthly plane, visible to everyone, realm of gross physical elements.

2. Your vital sheath exists in *sky realm*, intermediate plane of existence called "the void," sphere of subtle matter. This realm is said to extend from earth to the sun.

3. Your mental sheath resides in *subtle realm*, sphere of the great void, beyond gross and subtle matter. This plane is believed to extend from the sun to the polestar.

4. Your intellect sheath is in *middle region*, world of balance, beginning of illusion, connecting link or doorway between the spiritual and material world.

5. Your ego, which is part of your intellect sheath, lives in *place of rebirths*, where oneness separates into duality and individuality originates. It is called "the incomprehensible."

6. Your blissful sheath dwells in *mansion of the beloved*. This is also termed world of perfected beings, "the inaccessible," the unlimited sphere of the Holy Spirit.

7. Your higher self or atman is in *abode of truth*, the sphere of God, the only reality and only substance, the absolute. It is also called *anama*, "the nameless," because it is without form, time, or cause.

As we continue our journey to explore the power of auras, in the next chapter you will discover how science sees auras as they have researched subtle energy throughout the ages.

4

How Science Sees Auras

ཉཉ

Researching the Human Energy Field

"Give light and the darkness will disappear of itself."

—Erasmus[1]

Although the auric field and pranic energy are usually associated with the Orient, Western scientists or philosophers have also postulated an energy field permeating and surrounding the physical body. For example, after Newton published his laws of mechanics, optics, and gravity, he spent several years searching for the life-force through alchemy.

Most modern scientists either discount or ridicule the notion of an invisible energy body. However, scientific research verifying such an energy field is compelling. In this chapter you will discover researchers who advanced theories about the energy field. Many were persecuted or imprisoned for their beliefs.

Early Life-Energy Theories

Plato called it *nous* and Aristotle called it *entelecheia*. Hippocrates, the father of medicine, named it *vis medicatrix naturae:* "healing power of nature." To Pythagoras and Galen it was *pneuma*. The Greeks first proposed the concept of life energy in the West, and this tradition continued through the alchemists.

Philippus Theophrastus, known as Paracelsus (c. 1493–1541) believed that "the vital force is not enclosed in man but radiates within and around him like a luminous sphere."[2]

Johannes Kepler (1571–1630) termed this energy *vis motrix* ("life force"). Johann Baptista van Helmont (1577–1644), Belgian physician and alchemist, was first to propose animal magnetism or magnetic fluid, *magnale magnum,* a diffused, universal healing force, radiating from all humans.

Viennese doctor Franz Anton Mesmer (1734–1815), who lived in Paris, believed in magnetism, a mutual, reciprocal influence wielded by a universally diffused, incomparably subtle "fluid" that receives, propagates, and communicates all motor disturbances.

To learn more about these and other early researchers, and to see a chart listing many brave pioneers in the field of subtle energy research, read Chapter 4 of *The Power of Chakras.*

Using Vital Life Energy

The idea of harnessing life energy for healing has existed since Hippocrates. Modern scientists have postulated a dynamic energy that sustains and heals the human body.

Hahnemann: Dynamis

German physician Samuel Hahnemann (1755–1843), founder of homeopathy, who termed the universal spirit *dynamis,* viewed disease as a morbid misalignment with *Lebens-Erhaltungskraft* ("living principle"). Because he believed the cause of illness could never be known, diseases are classified by symptoms. An artificially produced resonant disease—a medicinal "potency" (homeopathic medicine) of similar symptoms—removes illness and stimulates the vital force to restore balance in the newly revived state of health.

Reichenbach: Odic Force

German industrialist, chemist, and inventor Baron Karl von Reichenbach (1788–1869) studied a cosmic force he termed *od, odylic,* or *odic* force. The word *Odic* is derived from *Wodan* (archaic German: "all-penetrating")—nature's unceasing power, a penetrating force that flows through everything.

Reichenbach's thousands of investigations on emanations from human bodies, magnets, plants, minerals, crystals, prisms, colors, heat, sunlight, moonlight, and chemical action found the odic field to be energetic, like a light wave, and also particulate, like a fluid. Conducted at great distances by all substances, it is charged or discharged by contact or proximity. Electropositive elements give people warm, unpleasant feelings. In contrast, electronegative elements produce cool, agreeable feelings.

Reichenbach discovered that the body's vital power has magnetic polarity. The left side of the body is negative and the right side is positive—a concept already known in Taoism, yoga, and acupuncture.

MacDougall: Soul-Substance

In the 19th century a Spiritualist measured the body weight of a dying man right before and right after death. The corpse weighed half an ounce less. All other theories summarily abandoned, the Spiritualist claimed that a soul weighs half an ounce.

In 1907 *American Medicine* reported that Duncan MacDougall, MD, of Haverhill, Massachusetts, replicated this experiment.[3] His first subject, a tuberculosis patient, lay on a bed built upon delicately balanced platform beam scales. For 220 minutes before death, the patient lost weight at the rate of 1 ounce per hour due to evaporation of sweat and moisture during respiration. The moment he expelled his last breath, the beam end suddenly dropped with a crash, hit the lower limiting bar, and remained without rebounding. The loss of weight was three-fourths of an ounce (21 grams).[4]

MacDougall's second and third patients both lost one and a half ounces at death. Another patient lost three-eighths of an ounce. MacDougall concluded that his patients lost something that he termed "soul-substance." Later MacDougall performed the same experiment on 15 dogs. They lost no perceptible weight at death.

In 1995, in another study at a Minneapolis Veteran's Hospital, all deceased individuals weighed exactly five-eighths of an ounce less than they did when alive.

Driesch: Vitalism

Hans Adolf Eduard Driesch (1867–1941), German philosophy professor and embryologist, discovered that a section of an early embryonic sea urchin could develop into a complete adult. Because this finding contradicted current mechanistic theories, it led him to the philosophy of Vitalism. This theory proposes a self-determining, invisible life-force—a "vital principle" or innate intelligence by which the body self-heals and self-regulates. Disease indicates disturbances in the vital force and induces reactions by the vital force. Vitalism supports and regulates the natural tendency to heal through diet, vitamins, exercise, healthy habits, eliminating toxins, and so on.

Inventing Energy Machines

Using the principles of life force energy, scientists developed machines to capture subtle energy as a power source or healing device. Tesla believed in "luminiferous ether," as did other inventors of energy machines.

Keely: Free Energy

American John Ernst Worrell Keely (1827–1898), inventor of the Keely motor, claimed to uncover the secret of "free energy"—drawn directly from *ether*, or space. In 1872 he filed his Hydro Vacuo Engine design with the U.S. Patent Office: "...an engine wherein the actuating power is produced by a vacuum in connection with water pressure."[5] Keely's key to free energy is controlling the incessant vibrations underlying all energies in the universe: "There is a celestial mind-force, a great sympathetic force which is life itself, of which everything is composed."[6] Keely's perpetual motion machine was on display for many years at The Franklin Institute in Philadelphia.

Reich: Orgone Energy

In the 1930s Dr. Wilhelm Reich (1897–1957), German-born psychiatrist and scientist, discovered bions and established biophysics. His *bions* are "basic life energy units" of *orgone*—pre-atomic "mass-free primordial power that operates throughout the universe as the basic life force."[7] Reich founded orgonomy, the study of life energy in all organisms, earth, atmosphere, and outer space.

Using high-quality optical microscopes with magnification of 2000x to 4000x, Reich observed energy fields of inanimate and animate objects, microorganisms, and human blood cells. He correlated orgone flow changes to physical and psychological disease and trauma.

Reich's orgone accumulator concentrated orgone energy to speed up natural healing. With the accumulator, he charged a vacuum discharge tube that conducted a current of electricity at a potential lower than its normal discharge potential.

Reich was imprisoned in Maine when charged by the Food and Drug Administration for transporting orgone accumulators over state lines. He died in prison a few months before his possible parole (only if he agreed never to work on or write about orgonomy again). No journals or personal items were ever released to his family. The United States FDA burned Reich's books in New York City at least twice—in the 1950s and 1960s.

Abrams: High Frequency Radiations

Pioneer of radionics, Albert Abrams, MD (1863–1924), posited that living organisms radiate and are affected by high frequency vibrations. He accurately identified and numerically classified specific resonant frequencies of pathogens with his diagnostic method, called Electronic Reaction of Abrams (E.R.A.).[8]

Abrams believed an invisible subtle body encompasses each individual. An etheric force field, linking all life, could serve as a medium to connect to patients. His "radiogeodiagnosis" proved effective for distance healing. His "telediagnosis" used telephone wires to link to patients, and "teleaerodiagnosis" connected to patients through nothing but the ethers.

A student of metaphysics, Dr. Abrams could unfailingly predict the hour and day of anyone's death, even his own, which he publicly predicted a year before his demise.

Drown and De La Warr: Radionics

American Ruth B. Drown, DC (1892–1963) and her colleague, British psychiatrist George De La Warr, MD (1904–1969), discovered that human body energy emissions could be photographed, even though their wavelengths differed from light.

Drown used her Homo-Vibra Ray Instrument to "broadcast" for distance treatment. In 1935 she upgraded this Radionic machine into an incredible camera that measured etheric life-energy body radiations and diagnosed and cured thousands of patients at a distance.[9] Using only hair samples of patients, it photographed tumors, cysts, cancer, and other diseases.[10]

Using a dried drop of blood on blotter paper, Drown photographed tissue anywhere in the body through a unique reverse method of film development. In 1960 her booklet for physicians displayed 22 stunning photographs: sharp images of various body organs, tissues, microbes, and tumors, shown in cross section (similar to CAT scans).[11]

Electromagnetic Auric Radiations

In the 1800s, with the discovery of the electromagnetic field, researchers sought to locate and measure an electric field emanating from the human body.

Burr, Northrop, and Ravitz: L-Fields

The Electrodynamic Theory of Life was developed by Dr. Harold Saxton Burr (1889–1973), embryologist and professor of neuroanatomy at Yale School of Medicine for 43 years, and Dr. F. S. C. Northrop, Sterling Professor of Philosophy and Law at Yale. Their theory revealed the basic blueprints of life: "electrodynamic fields" independent of matter, surrounding everything and interconnecting matter.[12]

In 1935 Burr, along with Dr. C. T. Land and Dr. L. F. Nims, perfected a voltmeter to measure electric currents of one millionth of a volt around organisms. In tens of thousands of experiments over 40 years, Burr and colleagues measured the "fields of life," or "L-fields."

Burr found that certain fields determine the structure, function, growth, shape, and decay of organisms, and that they disappear at death. These fields change in strength and polarity with emotions, sleep deprivation, narcosis, and hypnosis, and with lunar or seasonal cycles and the earth's magnetic field.

Dr. Leonard J. Ravitz, neuropsychiatrist with the Section of Neuroanatomy at Yale, related high voltage to irritability and tension, and low voltage to well-being and contentment. Burr proposed that doctors could diagnose illness before symptoms develop by measuring L-field voltages.

Puharich, Green, Zimmerman, and Seto: Biomagnetic Field

From 1960 to 1990 Dr. Andrija Puharich (1918–1995) found that during healing sessions, healers' hands produce a beneficial magnetic field of eight cycles per second (8 Hz).

In 1990 John Zimmerman, PhD, of the Bio-Electro-Magnetics Institute of Reno, Nevada, reported low-frequency biomagnetic fields around hands of Therapeutic Touch practitioners, measured by a magnetometer called SQUID (Superconducting Quantum Interference Device)—from 0.3 to 30 Hz, concentrating mostly in 7 to 8 Hz.[13]

In 1992 A. Seto of Japan used a magnetometer to measure biomagnetic fields from hands of meditators and practitioners of yoga and Qigong. These fields display the same range: 2 to 50 Hz.[14]

Healers' hands and earth's magnetic field pulse at the same rate: 8 Hz, known as the Schuman Resonance. Medical research has shown the low-frequency range stimulates bodily healing, with specific frequencies suitable for different tissues. Certain other frequencies are detrimental to life.

At the Menninger Clinic in 1993, physicist Dr. Elmer Green, pioneer of biofeedback, measured a dramatic voltage change spike, up to 220 volts induced onto a copper wall, from healers' hands while healing patients through focused intention.[15]

Becker: Electrical Control System

In 1962 Dr. Robert O. Becker MD, Professor of Orthopedic Surgery, Upstate Medical Center, Syracuse, New York, mapped a complex electrical field around the human body, shaped like the body and central nervous system. This field changes shape and strength with physiological and psychological changes. Continuing his research until 1979, he found particles the size of electrons moving through this field. Dr. Becker was nominated for the Nobel Prize for his pioneering work on the body's electrical control system.[16]

Motoyama: Energy Meridians

In the 1970s, Dr. Hiroshi Motoyama (b. 1925), author of more than 50 books and founder of the Institute of Religion and Psychology in Tokyo and the California Institute for Human Science in Encinitas, used a movie camera in a darkroom to measure low levels of light radiating from advanced yoga practitioners.

Motoyama's AMI Machine (Apparatus for Measuring the Functions of the Meridians and Corresponding Internal Organ), with 28 electrodes, acupuncture needles, or clips, electrically measures acupuncture meridians and pressure points. When Motoyama measured meridians of healers and patients before, during, and after treatment, usually the healer's energy dipped and then rose again. The energy in the heart area of healers increased after treatment.[17]

Sancier, Lin, and Jiang: Qi Energy

In 1996 considerable scientific evidence indicated that external qi emissions can alter the molecular structure of treated solutions; affect nucleotide polymerization, protein crystallization, and enzyme activity; increase the UV absorption of nucleic acids and catalyze chemical reactions; and alter the radioactive decay rate of a radioactive source by 1 to 12 percent.[18] These experiments were replicated from various locations, and the effects were identical when the subject and target were thousands of miles apart (United States to China, for example).

High-Frequency Photography

Since Kirlian first invented his photographic device in the early 1900s, researchers have been intrigued by the importance of Kirlian photography.

Kirlian: High-Frequency Photography

During an electrotherapy treatment, Semyon Davidovich Kirlian (1900–1980), technician at the Research Institute of Krasnodar in southern Russia near the Black Sea, noticed a tiny light flash between a high-frequency instrument's electrodes and the patient's skin.

In 1939 Kirlian discovered he could photograph the light emanations of organisms in a field of high-frequency electrical currents using a unique spark-generator of 75,000 to 200,000 cycles per second. A tree leaf, photographed by his method, revealed myriad dots of energy. Turquoise and reddish-yellow patterns flared from leaf veins. Kirlian's own hand resembled the Milky Way in a starry sky, with a fireworks display against a blue and gold background. Yet this pattern was unrelated to the hand's physiology.

This light-body appears intimately connected with the physical body and seems to direct its activities. Light patterns of healthy organisms differ widely from diseased organisms. Also, mental tension or emotional stress distort the patterns. By deciphering the photographs, Kirlian accurately diagnosed diseases long before symptoms appeared.

Soviet scientists, observing Kirlian photography, found that the flow of bioluminescence corresponds exactly to acupuncture meridians. Insertion points of acupuncture needles match precisely with brilliant flashes of light in Kirlian photographs.

As an organism dies, its bioluminescent energy-body oozes out. Its light intensity and orderliness reduce. Blobs of shimmering energy eject from the organism until eventually the bioluminescence disappears altogether at death.

Both animate and inanimate objects have been photographed using Kirlian's process. Inanimate objects are also permeated with biolumines-cent energy, but the light, which is of constant intensity, lacks the iridescence, movement, and animation of that in live organisms.

Moss: High-Voltage Photography

In the 1960s Dr. Thelma Moss (1918–1997) and her colleagues at the UCLA Neuropsychiatric Institute found that meditation, hypnosis, alcohol, drugs, or proximity to a close friend or person of the opposite sex induce a wider, more brilliant corona discharge on the fingertips in high-voltage, Kirlian-type photographs. In states of arousal, tension, or emotional excitement, researchers observed blotches on the color film.

At the UCLA Center for the Health Sciences, Moss and associates observed that after a hands-on healer treats a patient, the corona around the healer's fingertip diminishes, whereas the patient's corona becomes wider and more brilliant.

People claiming to have a "green thumb" with plants can increase the brightness of a mutilated leaf's corona by simply holding a hand above it for a few minutes. These leaves remain brighter for many weeks longer than control leaves. When subjects claiming to have a "brown thumb" try the same experiment, the leaf's corona disappears.

Studying the Bioplasmic Aura

The corona in Kirlian photographs was assumed to be electromagnetic. However, Inyushin of Kirov State University in Kazakhstan postulated that Kirlian's light is a new energy: *bioplasma,* a fifth state of matter. (The four others are solids, liquids, gases, and plasma.)

Inyushin and Korotkov: Bioplasma and Electrophotonics

Starting in the 1950s, biophysicist Dr. Victor M. Inyushin studied the bioplasmic energy field. He found bioplasmic bioluminescence is caused by orderly structured emissions of ionized free atomic protons and electrons. Bioplasmic particles are constantly renewed by cellular chemical processes. A severe shift in the balance of positive and negative particles indicates disease. The bioplasmic body emanates its own electromagnetic field, changing with emotional moods and influenced by other fields. Breathing oxygen charges and replenishes the bioplasmic body.[19]

After 20 years of research, physicist Konstantin G. Korotkov (b. 1952), at St. Petersburg State Technical University in Russia, developed the Gas Discharge Visualization (GDV). His system of Electrophotonics creates stunning, real-time photos and videos of humans, organisms, water, and gems. The GDV device reports potential health abnormalities prior to earliest symptoms, and suggests remedies. In his words, Kirlian photography is like a bicycle, while his camera is like a Mercedes. His technology is widely accepted throughout Russia and Europe.

Popov Group: Bioplasmic Body

Under the direction of Professor Ippolite M. Kogan, from 1965 to 1975, Soviet scientists from the Bioinformation Institute of A. S. Popov All-Union Scientific and Technical Society of Radio Technology and Electrical Communications extensively researched ESP and telepathy. They found that living organisms emit VLF (very low frequency) or ELF (extremely low frequency) electromagnetic waves at a frequency of 300 to 2,000 nanometers.

This biofield or bioplasma becomes stronger in subjects more successful at transferring their bioenergy. Telepathic messages and psychic perceptions are conveyed through the bioplasmic body. The biofield changes when subjects receive telepathy. Stimulation of chakra and *marma* points (points where concentrated prana is located, according to Ayurveda) in the bioplasmic body increases psychic awareness.[20]

Measuring Biophotons

Since the pioneering days of Soviet scientists, researchers have measured light emanating from organisms. Popp of Germany termed these emissions biophotons.

Popp, Cohen, and Colleagues: Biophotons

Since 1972 German-born Dr. Fritz-Albert Popp (b. 1938), of the International Institute of Biophysics in Neuss, Germany, has extensively researched biophotons (biological quantum radiations) with a unique, supersensitive measuring device.

In 1976 Popp and B. Ruth (a physicist at Marburg University) measured permanent light emissions (400 to 800 nanometers) from plant and animal cells and tissues.[21] In 1981 Popp found evidence of DNA as a biophoton source and speculated that DNA may store and release virtual photons in the cells as energy, and transmit biophotonic emissions as information within and between cells.[22] From 1981 to 1999, Popp studied coherence of the biophoton field[23] and intra- and intercellular biocommunication through biophotons.[24] In 1997 Popp and French-born Sophie Cohen (b. 1968) discovered that biophotons indicate human biological rhythms and that various diseases disrupt normal biophoton patterns.[25]

Ronliang, Wallace, and Nakamara: Qigong Emissions

In the 1990s, at Shanghai Atomic Nuclear Institute of Academia in Sinica, China, Dr. Zheng Ronliang of Lanzhou University, using a leaf vein connected to a photo quantum device, found that a Qigong master's hands emit a "vital force" with "a very low [frequency] fluctuating carrier wave."[26] Sometimes qi is detected as a micro-particle flow with particle diameter of 60 microns and velocity of 20 to 50 centimeters per second.[27]

In 1999 Dr. Eugene Wallace reported measurements of 100 times stronger biophoton emissions from the hands of gifted Qigong practitioners. Using a solid-state photon counting device, Wallace found that "more photons were measured" when people "intended to emit more energy."[28]

In 2000 Nakamura and colleagues found hands of Qigong practitioners during Qigong dropped in surface temperature and increased in biophoton emission intensity.[29]

Measuring Gamma Ray Emissions

A recent theory in biophoton research is that high-energy gamma photons are digested, stored, and used as an energy source by human cells.

Luckey and Slawinski: Radiogenic Metabolism

In 1980 cellular biologist Dr. T. D. Luckey introduced the theory of "radiogenic metabolism": "the promotion of metabolic reactions by ionizing radiation and its products," which involves "prephotosynthetic transformation of radiant energy into chemical energy."[30] A by-product of low-energy photon emissions would suggest that radiogenic metabolism exists. Many researchers have detected such emissions, ranging from ultraviolet to near infrared (200 to 900 nanometers).

In 1987 biophysicist Dr. Janusz Slawinski found that "all dying cell populations and organisms emit a radiation 10 to 1,000 times stronger than their stationary emission during homeostasis. That phenomenon... called a 'light shout,' is universal and independent of the cause of death. Its intensity and time course reflect the rate of dying."[31]

Benford: Gamma Radiation

In 1999 M. Sue Benford, RN, measured a significant decrease in gamma radiation levels in polarity therapists during sessions: "Gamma radiation levels markedly decreased during therapy sessions of 100% of subjects and at every body site tested."[32]

Similar results were found in 1996 by Dr. Elmer Green, who measured unexplainable "body-potential surges of negative polarity ranging from 4 volts to 190 volts" in non-contact therapeutic touch therapists.[33]

Gamma rays, often called cosmic radiation, are highly energetic forms of light, which, theoretically, should not be influenced by human bodies. Yet a substantial decrease in gamma radiation during healing sessions indicates that gamma radiation is absorbed, metabolized, and stored by the human cells as an alternative energy source.[34]

Environmental Auric Influences

The life-energy force-field is not confined to the human body. Scientists envision this energy as fundamental to all organisms and linking all of life. Researchers have attempted to define and measure this extended energy field.

Strömberg: Genii

In 1940 Swedish cosmologist and Mount Wilson astronomer Gustaf Strömberg (1882–1962) postulated a complex network of organizational waves, or *genii* (sing. *genie*), which, though entirely nonmaterial, direct material particles and the structural development of organisms. Some genii function as memory accumulators, such as changing larvae into butterfly or dividing and reproducing cells.[35] Strömberg conceived a world-enveloping genie, the "World Soul," as well as genii governing chromosomal genes, called *gene-spirits*. His work was favorably reviewed by Einstein and Eddington.

Hall and Sommer: Personal Space

In the 1960s researchers investigated "personal space"—the comfort zone of interpersonal proximity. In 1969 E. T. Hall delineated four zones: intimate, personal, social, and public. Less than one meter is considered intimate or personal space zones. He found that comfort zones vary by situation, culture, individuals, and sex.[36]

In R. Sommer's 1969 studies, researchers invaded the personal space of target subjects who were sitting alone in libraries by approaching these subjects at various distances. They then recorded the closeness in distance and the rapidity of time before the subject moved away.[37] In 1969, Hall reported that, when personal space is violated, the person might withdraw, avoid further social contact, make postural changes, move away, talk less, avoid eye contact, or increase personal distance.[38]

Maharishi Mahesh Yogi: Collective Influences

More than 500 scientific studies show the effects of Transcendental Meditation (TM) and TM-Sidhi program of Maharishi Mahesh Yogi (1918–2008), who proposed a pervasive field of collective consciousness (mass influence of individuals comprising a society) of harmony or disharmony, which reciprocally affects each individual. Extensive research confirms that increasing the number of meditators in a city improves quality of life.

From 1974 to 1978, a study of 160 U.S. cities showed significant reduction in crime directly proportional to the number of people in each city who had learned the TM technique by 1973. More TM meditators in any given population result in fewer homicides, suicides, and traffic fatalities, and reduced crime, unemployment, and inflation. When a sufficiently large group meditates at the same time in the same city, international relations improve and regional conflicts decrease worldwide.[39]

Bohm: Causal Quantum Theory

American quantum physicist David Joseph Bohm (1917–1992) proposed a ubiquitous "quantum potential" directly linking quantum systems, providing "active information" about the whole environment. Because of this cosmic quantum field, whatever happens in one part of the universe immediately affects the motion of particles at the other end of the cosmos. He stated that his Causal Quantum Theory "opens the door for the creative operation of underlying, and yet subtler, levels of reality."[40]

In 1959, with research student Yakir Aharonov, Bohm discovered that in certain circumstances electrons "feel" the presence of a nearby magnetic field even while traveling in regions of space where the field strength is zero. This is called the Aharonov-Bohm Effect.

Sheldrake: Morphogenetic Fields

In 1995 British biologist Rupert Sheldrake (b. 1942) postulated that energy fields called "morphogenetic fields" unite entities—even human and non-human. He proposed that the morphogenetic field underlying the universe is consciousness.[41] Sheldrake defined a "morphic unit" as a unit of form or organization, such as an atom, molecule, crystal, organism, cell, plant, animal, social group, instinctive behavioral pattern, cultural element, ecosystem, planet, planetary system, or galaxy.

In Sheldrake's hypothesis of "formative causation," the structure and activity of morphic units are organized by "morphic fields," including morphogenetic, behavioral, social, cultural, and mental fields. Morphic fields are shaped, influenced, and stabilized by "morphic resonance," an increasingly habitual collective memory from all previous similar morphic units.

Through morphic resonance, formative causal influences traverse space and time without losing strength. The power of influence of morphic resonance is directly proportional to the degree of similarity with previous morphic units.

In 2002, through extensive double-blind studies, Sheldrake found that dogs can ascertain in advance when their masters will return home.[42] In 2003 he also established that humans know when other people are staring at them.[43] These studies appear to validate his theory of morphic resonance.

In the next chapter you will open your awareness to subtle sense perception, whereby you can begin to feel, sense, and see auras.

Part II

୬୯

Experiencing Your Energy Field

5

You Can See and Feel Energy

ﮯ

Experiencing Subtle Vibrations

"It isn't more light we need, it's putting into practice what light we already have."

—Peace Pilgrim[1]

Can you often tell how people are really feeling, even though they act differently? Have you ever noticed when someone is staring at you? Can you tell when someone is nearby before you actually see that person? Do certain people have a draining effect on you? If you answered yes to any of these questions, then you are sensitive to subtle energy and have already experienced auric fields.

Feeling an aura is more common than seeing one. That is because most people are more clairsentient than clairvoyant, and seeing auras with clarity requires a high degree of clairvoyant aptitude. In any case, you can perceive auras through any of your five subtle senses: sight, hearing, taste, touch, or smell.

Through the sense of touch, you undoubtedly get gut feelings about people and places. Your first impression of a person is sensing a subtle auric field, which you can read, often with great accuracy. We speak of seeing someone's true colors. Rarely does this involve clairvoyant sight to "see" colors; rather, it means sensing true motives.

Few people have the rare skill of outer clairvoyance, whereby they clearly see colors in auras with their eyes open. However, many people see colors and other details of auras through inner clairvoyant vision, with eyes closed.

In this chapter you will practice simple exercises to help you see, feel, sense, and experience auric energy. These exercises are easy to do, and you might be surprised when results come instantly. It is best to have no particular expectations—neither positive nor negative—going into the experiments. Most people take months or years to develop "second sight" or clairvoyant vision. So, if you do not get immediate results, be patient with yourself. You might find some experiments are more successful than others.

Developing clairvoyance is a lifelong study that often requires personal habits of mental and physical purity and a wholesome lifestyle. With a sincere desire to heal yourself and to lift others, you can succeed.

How to Feel Subtle Energy

This world of vibrations is filled with subtle energies. You are a vibratory being moving through these frequencies, picking up energies. In fact, you are already sensitive to the subtle energy called prana or chi. Here are some examples:

What do you feel when you enter a hospital, prison, bar, mental institution, or crowded bus? Do you get a sickening sensation or feel energy drain? If so, then you can sense detrimental vibrations. Have you ever felt elated by hiking in the woods, boating on a lake, hearing inspiring music, or reading uplifting poetry or scriptures? If you have, then you can feel beneficial vibrations.

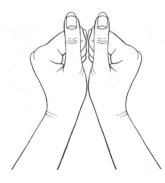

Figure 5a. Energy Sphere

Later in this book you will learn to energize your body, enhance your energy field, heal energy blockages, and prevent energy drain. Here are a few experiments to help you become more sensitive to subtle energies:

Buffing Up

Clench both your fists and place them next to each other, as shown in Figure 5a. Vigorously rub your fists against each other for 45 seconds in a buffing, washboard motion. Then unclench your fists and face your palms toward each other a few inches apart. Slowly move your palms in and out. You might feel an invisible ball of energy between your palms. A sense of pressure, tickling, prickling, thickness, warmth, or cooling may arise. This vibrant activity is the subtle energy called *prana*.

Feeling Energy Vortices

Sit comfortably, close your eyes, and take deep breaths. Imagine energy building in the index finger of your dominant hand (right finger if you are right-handed; left finger if you are left-handed). Once you sense energy in your index finger, then open your eyes and point your index finger about 3 to 6 inches away from your non-dominant hand's open palm. Rotate your index finger in small circles while imagining a stream of spiraling energy vortex drilling into your non-dominant hand's palm. You might sense warmth, coolness, prickling, or tingling in your palm. You may even feel a "hole" in your palm.

Creating Auric Vortices

Stand behind a friend's back. Close your eyes, take some deep breaths, and imagine energy building up in your dominant hand's index finger. Point your index finger 6 to 12 inches from your friend's back. Create an energy vortex by rotating your index finger and imagining energy streaming from your fingertip. Visualize your fingertip boring into your friend's energy field. After you have created a hole in your friend's aura, ask your friend to identify where you have been pointing.

Then draw a simple diagram, such as a circle, square, or triangle, on your friend's auric field about 6 to 12 inches away from his/her physical body. Continue to trace over the diagram repeatedly until the shape is "engraved" into your friend's aura. Then ask your friend to identify and locate the shape.

Pushing the Auric Egg

This exercise is done with three people. Stand behind person A's back. Ask person B to observe. Imagine an egg-shaped sphere around person A. Extend your hands toward person A and shove the imaginary eggshell, as though trying to topple it over. Then pull on the eggshell and bring it toward you. Push strongly. Then pull strongly. Continue to push and pull. Move in a slow, intensely concentrated fashion. Person A's energy field will move, and he or she will begin to sway backward and forward. Person B will notice this swaying motion.

Sensing Personal Space

Ask a friend to close his or her eyes and stand still while you walk toward him/her and then report at what point he/she feels uncomfortable. Do this while approaching from the front, side, and back. Then repeat the process as your friend approaches you. Through this exercise you can map your personal space and get a sense of auric intrusions.

Awakening Subtle Vision

In 1970 Cambridge biologist Oscar Bagnall proposed that auras are viewed with rods—sensory neurons on the side of the retina, responsible for night vision. So auras are more easily viewed with peripheral vision, out of the corner of the eye, rather than focusing hard and looking directly at them. Bagnall described two sections of the aura, observed through screens stained with dicyanin dyes. He found people in robust health have brighter auras with sharper outlines.[2]

It is quite easy to see light surrounding living things. After mastering seeing light, you will start to see colors. Here are some exercises to help you see subtle light.

Accessing Peripheral Vision

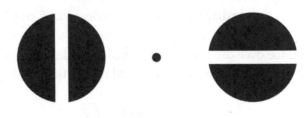

Figure 5b. Eye Exercise

Place the diagram in Figure 5b about 2 feet in front of your eyes. Take off your glasses, if you wear them. Concentrate intensely at the dot between the two circles for 60 seconds. Focus attention only on that one exact point. Meanwhile, your peripheral vision will automatically see the two large circles. After a few seconds, you will see a white edge surrounding the two large circles. This exercise stimulates peripheral vision capacity, which is useful for seeing auras.

Make a similar diagram out of colored paper, with one red circle and one green circle, or one blue and one orange. As you concentrate on the dot in the center, a "halo" of light of the opposite color will surround the circles.

Remember this exercise, because the halo or afterimage effect appears as any given color's compliment. Thus, when viewing auras, you might think someone wearing a red dress has a green aura, but it is the afterimage of the dress—not the aura of the person.

Gazing With Soft Focus

In order to see auras, it is essential to see with soft focus. That means gazing at an object or person without focusing intently at any one point. If you can pick out objects from embedded pictures, then you have mastered the art of seeing with soft focus.

Place Figure 5b about 2 feet in front of your eyes. Rather than looking at the center point intently, now gaze at the entire diagram as though looking at an embedded picture. Allow your eyes to relax. Eventually your eyes will per-

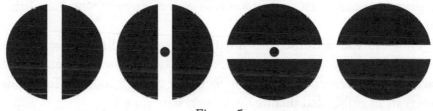

Figure 5c.

ceive Figure 5b as though it looks like Figure 5c, with four circles and two dots.

Continue to gaze at the entire diagram in Figure 5b, without blinking, until you perceive only three circles and two dots with a cross in the center,

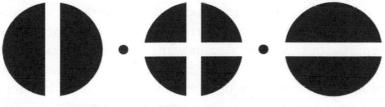

Figure 5d.

as shown in Figure 5d.

One of the circles will appear to cover the other one. The circle with the vertical line represents the brain's right hemisphere. The circle with the horizontal line symbolizes the left hemisphere. Depending on your dominant hemisphere, you will see that circle cover the other one. Now continue to gaze at Figure 5b until the hidden circle dominates.

Now gaze at Figure 5b further until you perceive the cross is made perfectly balanced without one circle dominating the other. This powerful exercise stimulates your brain and creates coherence between your right- and left-brain hemispheres. Five minutes of this exercise doubles your bio-energy. It is an excellent warm-up before practicing on "real" subjects.

Seeing Auras Is Normal

Seeing colors is considered normal for sighted people. Yet, to the visually challenged, ordinary colors do not exist. Those who are blind to the auric field also have a disability. For seeing auric colors is as normal as seeing colors through the eyes. We are all born to perceive subtle energies.

Some people see auras better with their eyes open; others see or sense auras better with their eyes closed. If you belong to the latter category, you can learn to read auras as well as anyone who "sees" them clairvoyantly.

How can you rekindle your innate clairvoyant ability? Observing the aura is a hide-and-seek game. Rather than staring intensely, observe the space around the person with soft focus, as though looking for hidden objects in an embedded picture. Stay alert, without effort.

As with any other skill in life, practice is the key to accomplishment. Here are a few exercises to help you develop this skill.

Seeing Energy Fields in Nature

Lie on your back outdoors on a warm, sunny day. Relax and gaze at trees or bushes in the distance. Let your eyes move up and down the trees and then notice the line where the treetops meet the sky. Gaze at the treetops with soft focus. A faint white halo will appear around the trees. Now look at buildings in the distance. You may perceive a narrow band of light, but it will not be as vibrant or as large as the aura of the trees.

Seeing the Aura of Your Hand

In dim light, hold your own hand at arm's length against a neutral colored background. Take deep breaths and relax. Stare intently at a fingertip or a space between your fingers for about 30 seconds. Then suddenly shift your focus. Gaze at the space around your hand with soft focus. You might see a band of white light outlining the hand. Rays and streamers of color may radiate from your fingers.

Seeing Fingertip Energy

Sit down, close your eyes, and relax. Take deep breaths. Touch the fingertips of one hand with the fingertips of the other hand for two minutes, while continuing in a meditative state. Then open your eyes, look at your hands with soft focus, and slowly draw your fingertips apart. You might perceive auric radiations emanating from the fingertips.

Seeing an Aura

View your subject in dim lighting against a neutral background. The aura of a public speaker on a stage against a white screen or wall is easily visible. However, if the person is standing before a bright-colored, multi-colored, or patterned background, your perception of the aura color might be distorted.

If possible, view your subject indoors with light falling evenly on the subject. Natural daytime light is better than artificial light. Candlelight is okay as long as shadows are not cast on the background. Fluorescent light and direct sunlight are not recommended. If it is daytime, ask the person to stand opposite a window.

Sit facing the subject about 10 feet away. Ask the subject to breathe deeply, exhale fully, and relax. Close your own eyes, relax, take deep breaths, and become quiet, centered, and directed inward. Imagine the subject's aura with your inner vision for a few moments.

Open your eyes, and take off your glasses if you wear them. When looking at the subject, rather than staring directly, gaze with soft focus at the forehead, above the head, the curve of the neck, or past the head and shoulders toward the background. Relax and allow light to enter your eyes rather than grasping or focusing sharply.

Notice any mist, light, rays, or colors emanating from the body. You might see a white, gray, silver, or clear band of light about 1 or 2 inches wide, right next to the body. A light may shine behind the head, pointing upward. Or perhaps electricity swirls around the body. You may not see these emanations, but you may feel or sense them.

Then close your eyes again. Relax. Take deep breaths. Then return to observing. This time, gaze at the outer edge of the white band. Relax as you alternately close your eyes, take deep breaths, and view the aura again. After some practice, flashes or dots of color will appear.

Here are some more pointers:

- Concentrate intently on the subject's forehead for 30 to 60 seconds. Then shift your focus to become soft. Widen your gaze to encompass the subject's entire body.

- Look at the subject's forehead. Then rapidly draw several circles with your eyes around the person's body, first clockwise, then counterclockwise. This will stimulate the rods and cones in your eyes.

- "Frame" the subject's face with your hands, with your thumb tips touching and index fingers pointing upward (as though they were two "L's" facing each other). Gaze at the subject's forehead with soft focus while simultaneously moving your hands apart slowly. Allow your peripheral vision to follow your hands.

- Ask the subject to dress in white clothing against a white background to overcome false afterimage effects.

- Ask the subject to think of something he/she is excited about or upset about. This can bring more visible colors into the aura.

- Ask the subject to speak about something with deep meaning— about life purpose or plans for the future. More vibrations or colors may appear in the aura.

- Gaze out the window at the sky (not the sun) for a minute before observing auras. Or, if it is nighttime, gaze at an electric light bulb for a minute.

- Ask the person to rock from side to side. Observe whether the aura moves when the body moves.

Feeling an Aura

Stand about 3 feet from the subject. Ask the subject to breathe deeply, relax, and keep his/her eyes closed. Close your own eyes, relax, take deep breaths, and become quiet, centered, and directed inward. Then open your eyes. Place your hands approximately 6 to 12 inches away from the subject's body. Notice whether you feel greater energy near the top of the head, the heart, the solar plexus, or the sacral area. Notice whether any places in the energy field feel "stuck." Sense whether any areas seem healthy and vibrant or depleted and drained. Ask the subject to open his/her eyes and share what you experienced.

Seeing an Aura With Eyes Closed

Ask someone to sit about 3 feet in front of you. Sit comfortably, close your eyes, take a few deep breaths, and enter a relaxed, meditative state along with the person. Now ask your higher self to show you the subject's energy field. Take a few more deep breaths and let go. Do not open your eyes. Simply observe what you "see" with your inner vision. You may sense colors, objects, anomalies, energies, or thought-forms (crystallized patterns of energy created by thoughts, habits, and beliefs) in the person's energy field. Tell the person what you are sensing. Ask for feedback. Continue this process until it feels complete. Then take deep breaths and come out of meditation. Share what you have experienced.

Seeing Your Aura in a Mirror

You can see your own aura by gazing into a mirror in dim light as you stand or sit about 2 feet away from the mirror against a white or neutral background. Gaze at your forehead or the curve of your own neck with soft focus, and you will begin to see a white band around your body. Observe and rest alternately, while breathing deeply, until you begin to see flashes of light and color.

Seeing Group Auric Radiations

Place a non-shiny black cloth on a table, and sit with several friends. Everyone then rests hands on the table with palms downward. Ask everyone to close their eyes, take deep breaths, and get centered for a few minutes. Then you all open your eyes. Keeping your hands on the table, point your fingers toward a friend's fingers. With soft focus, you might see or sense radiations uniting your fingers with your friend's fingers. A dark line may appear between the fingers and the aura surrounding them. The aura from all the hands might join in the center like a luminous cloud of rapidly moving particles.

Developing Inner Sensitivity

The following experiments are easy, fun projects that can help you develop sensitivity to subtle energies and auric fields.

Sensing Crystals and Magnets

Place a very large crystal and/or magnet in an absolutely dark room (or under the covers in bed). Relax for three minutes, and become quiet, still, and serene. Gaze steadily at each object with soft focus. The magnet's poles may emanate a faint, pale, hazy patch of light or clearly defined rays. The crystal's point may glow with fine, streaming, tulip-shaped blue light, continually in motion, emitting sparks, and disappearing in fine vapor. A dense red and yellow smoke may rise from the crystal's back end.

Turn on the lights and place the palm of your left hand within 3 to 6 inches from each end of the crystal. What feeling emanates from each end of the crystal? A fine, cool, pleasant, refreshing current may flow from the crystal's point. Yet, from its back end, you might get a lukewarm, unpleasant, tiring sensation.

Feeling Color Vibrations

Use a large prism to split sunlight onto a wall. Or use a high-tech alternative: Place a flat color onto a PowerPoint slide on your computer and project a beam from a projector. Then hold your left hand in various colored light beams so the light shines onto your palm. Notice how you feel when you isolate each color.

When the color is refracted into blue or violet, you may notice a pleasant coolness, purer and cooler than an unrefracted sunbeam. When the color is yellow or red, you might feel heat, discomfort, or nausea, and your arm may feel heavy.

Sensing Hand Polarities

Place your left hand in your friend's left hand and your right hand in your friend's right hand. Hold hands for five minutes. Then place your right hand in your friend's left hand and your left hand in your friend's right hand. Hold hands for five minutes. What differences do you feel?

You may notice that when you hold the same hands, you feel a disagreeable, lukewarm sensation. When you hold opposite hands, you may feel a pleasant, cool sensation.

Feeling Polarities of Touch

With your right hand, touch the left side of your friend's head, your friend's left shoulder, left arm, left side, left hip, left leg, left knee, and left foot. Then, with your right hand, touch the right side of your friend's head, your friend's right shoulder, right arm, right side, right hip, right leg, right knee, and right foot. Then share how you felt.

You may find that when you touch the left side of the body

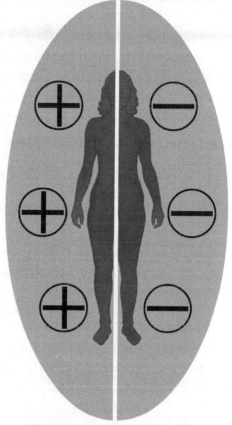

Figure 5e. Energy Polarities

with your right hand, there is an enjoyable, pleasant, cooling sensation, but, when you touch the right side of the body with your right hand, the sensation is uncomfortable, lukewarm, and nauseating.

Feeling Side-to-Side Polarities

Stand beside a friend, with your right shoulder touching your friend's left shoulder, for three minutes. Then turn around so your left shoulder touches your friend's left shoulder for three minutes. Share how you felt in these positions.

You may notice that when opposite shoulders touched, you felt a comfortable, cooling, pleasant sensation. Yet when the same shoulders touched, you felt uncomfortable, off-balance, and nauseated.

Feeling Back-to-Front Polarities

Stand just behind a friend so the front of your body snuggles up against your friend's back. Stay there for one minute. Then stand back-to-back for another minute, and front-to-front (hugging) for another minute. Then compare your feelings.

You might notice that when you are front-to-front or back-to-back, you feel a cool, pleasant, agreeable sensation. But when you snuggle front-to-back, you feel an unpleasant, lukewarm, nauseating, off-balance feeling.

Sensing Polarity Energies

Sit beside a friend, with your left shoulder touching your friend's right shoulder, for five minutes. Then switch positions. (Your right shoulder now touches your friend's left shoulder for five minutes.) Then share what both of you felt.

When you sit to the right of your friend, you may notice an agreeable, cooling sensation, as though you were gaining energy. When you sit to the left, you might feel a warming, disagreeable, nauseating, draining feeling.

In the next chapter, you will learn new ways to experience and measure the human energy field by using L-rods and pendulums.

6

How Big Is Your Aura?

ཨེ

Mapping and Measuring Energy Fields

"There is not enough darkness in all the world to put out the light of even one small candle."

—Robert Alden[1]

Perhaps you are one of those gifted clairvoyants who can see auras clearly—or maybe not. For those who are less than clairvoyant, this chapter is indispensable. Even with no clairvoyant abilities whatsoever, here you will practice simple, ancient methods for "seeing" auras without the benefit of supernormal sight.

In 1949, while searching for evidence of lost civilizations, French explorers discovered an 8,000-year-old cave painting at Tassili-n-Ajjer in the foothills of the Atlas Mountains of Algeria, in the Sahara Desert. This painting shows a man holding a forked stick surrounded by fellow tribesmen. This archeological find reveals that the art of *dowsing*, or divining, has existed for thousands of years.

Today dowsing can locate wells, mineral deposits, oil, buried treasure, archaeological artifacts, lost items, and even missing people. However, an unknown fact is that it can measure, heal, and amplify energy fields of individuals and atmospheres. In this book you will learn to use specific dowsing tools for this purpose.

Dowsing History Highlights

Early evidence of the art of dowsing is found in many cultures. The Cairo Museum displays ceramic pendulums from 1,000-year-old tombs. Etchings on a 4,000-year-old Egyptian temple wall depict pharaohs holding rods, called *Ur-Heka* (the great magical power). Cleopatra employed two full-time dowsers who searched for gold.

In China, in an etching from the Xia Dynasty (2205–1766 BC), Emperor Yu holds a bulky pronged device. The Hebrews, Scythians, Persian Medes, Etruscans, Druids, Greeks, Romans, Hindus, Polynesians, Arabian tribes, Peruvians, and Native American Indians all used rods or wands. In the Bible Moses and Aaron located water springs with rods.

The blind Greek poet Homer coined the term *rhabdomancy*, from the roots *rhabdos* ("rod") and *manteia* ("diviner" or "prophet"), to describe the art of locating underground water or precious metals. Dowsing was widely practiced in Crete as early as 400 BC. The Pytheon Oracle of Delphi used a pendulum to answer questions posed by kings, queens, nobility, and military commanders, who traveled great distances to confer with her.

In 16th- and 17th-century Europe, dowsers, who used rods widely to locate coal deposits, were denounced as practitioners of evil. Martin Luther (1483–1546), leader of the Protestant Reformation in Germany, condemned dowsing as "the work of devil." He issued a proclamation declaring that using the rod violated the First Commandment. The term "water witching" was coined.

In India pendulums have been used for hundreds of years. However, the first illustrations of pendulums in the West were engraved on the side of wooden axe hafts used by miners' guilds in Saxony between 1664 and 1749.

Marines stationed in Vietnam used pendulums to locate underground mines, ammunition dumps, tunnels, and enemy movements. During World War II, pendulums helped British Intelligence outwit Hitler by predicting his next move.

L'Abbé Bouly (1865–1958), a French priest, coined the term *radiesthesia*, derived from the Latin *radius* ("radiance") and the Greek *aesthesis* ("sensitivity"), to describe pendulum use for detecting and measuring all radiations from minerals, plants, animals, or humans, whether magnetic, electromagnetic, or other unknown energies.

After World War I another Frenchman, Abbé Alexis Mermet (1866–1937), Rector of Chapelle de Sainte-Madeleine, was acclaimed as the "King of Pendulumists" throughout Europe. The Pope and the Vatican sought his help for archaeological research in Rome. With psychic radiesthesia, he discovered petroleum fields in Africa, Galicia, and other areas at a distance. He also located water and coal and traced missing relatives.

In 1922 American Dr. Albert Abrams (1863–1924) published a book about detecting and treating disease with medical radiesthesia. He found that the human body is a kind of broadcasting station that projects high-frequency radiations from every cell, tissue, and organ.

André Bovis, French professional wine-and-cheese taster, detected the quality and freshness of foods and measured magnetic currents with a pendulum. He found that the earth has positive magnetic currents running north to south, and negative magnetic currents running east to west. He discovered that humans are affected by these lines of force, and that vibratory currents emanate from human bodies.

Bovis developed a device called a *biometer* to measure the intensity of rays emanating from any place, plant, or object using the *angstrom* as a unit. Later, physicist André Simoneton changed the name to *bovis unit*. The biometer measures from 0 to 18,000 units with 6,500 as neutral point. The center of the labyrinth in the cathedral of Chartres near Paris was measured at the value 18,000.

Nobel Laureate Dr. Alexis Carrel (1873–1944), celebrated pioneer in surgery and organ transplants, studied the pendulum under auspices of the Rockefeller Institute of New York. He concluded that, for physicians, "radiesthesia is worthy of serious consideration."[2]

Albert Einstein found dowsing to be fascinating and believed electromagnetism would give scientific answers about why it works. He stated, "I know very well that many scientists consider dowsing as they do astrology, as a type of ancient superstition. According to my conviction this is, however, unjustified. The dowsing rod is a simple instrument which shows the reaction of the human nervous system to certain factors which are unknown to us at this time."[3]

Intuitive Kinesiology

I have coined the name *Intuitive Kinesiology* to describe the methods you will learn in this chapter. This term consists of *intuitive*, which means "inner knowing" or "insight," and *kinesiology*, which means "the study of movement."

Intuitive Kinesiology is a branch of knowledge that studies the movements of various tools that develop and enhance intuition. Some of these tools are muscle-testing or muscle-checking, dowsing, divining, and radiesthesia.

Intuitive Kinesology is defined as a quest for hidden information with or without an instrument (such as L-rod or pendulum), through knowing without conscious use of reason. It helps you access your inner source of knowledge and use this intuitive information for the highest good. Because this vast field of knowledge cannot be adequately covered here, in this book you will learn just a few simple tools to measure and enhance the size, strength, and health of energy fields.

Learning Intuitive Kinesiology is no more mysterious than your own internal sensory apparatus, whereby you see, hear, taste, smell, and feel. This "sixth sense" is natural to everyone, and it can be developed with a little practice.

Intuitive Kinesiology tools and techniques are communication, interface, or read-out devices controlled by your own higher mind or higher self. Before you begin any of these practices, I strongly suggest you take time for the following cautionary preparations:

Warm-Up Exercises

1. First, drink a full glass of fresh water.

2. Find a quiet place where you can be alone and comfortable.

3. Turn to page 236 of this book and practice the Energy Warm-Up Exercises.

4. Turn to page 238 of this book and practice the Brain Gym exercises.

5. Take some deep breaths, relax, and become quiet. Drift into a prayerful mood.

6. Speak aloud the Self-Authority Affirmation on page 159 of this book for spiritual self-defense and divine protection.

7. Speak a prayer or simply state your intention for your session audibly. Here is a possible example, but you can use your own words:

I recognize that there is one power and one presence in the universe, God the good, omnipotent. God is the source of wisdom. God is clarity and precision. God is perfection everywhere now. I AM one with this God source. My mind is filled with the wisdom, clarity, and precision of God now. I AM an instrument of divine power and glory now. I therefore claim my perfect Intuitive Kinesiology session now, which proceeds perfectly with divine order and timing. I now know that my questions are formed with clarity. My hands are guided by inner divinity. My mind is attuned to divine wisdom. My intuition and sensitivity are clear. My purpose for this session is blessed for the highest good for all concerned. I AM an instrument of God as I now fulfill the goal of this session. Thank you God and SO IT IS.

8. Before asking your inquiry, first ask your higher self for permission. If another person is involved, get permission from that individual before proceeding. Getting permission involves the following:

    1) May I?—Do I have permission to find this target?
    2) Can I?—Am I capable of successfully finding this target, and am I ready to proceed?
    3) Is it highest wisdom?—Is it appropriate for me to find this target, or would it not be wise at this time?

    Here is one way to word your permission question:
    "Do I have permission to [look for this particular target, ask this particular question]?"

9. Take more deep breaths and center yourself in an alert, relaxed state. Now you are ready to proceed.

Important Note: Do not attempt any exercises or experiments in this chapter until you drink adequate water and complete the suggested Warm-Up Exercises.

How to Use L-Rods

Every Intuitive Kinesiology tool has a Ready position, a Yes position, a No position, a Found position, a Line of Bearing position, a Clearing position, and an Increasing position.

The Ready position is a neutral position where you are ready to use your tool to ask a question or find a target. The Line of Bearing position indicates the direction where the target will be found or in which direction energy is flowing. The Yes position designates the answer to your question is yes. The No position shows your answer is no. The Found position confirms that you have found the specified target, such as a hidden object, lost object, underground stream, ley line, detrimental zone, or outer edge of an auric field. The Clearing position indicates that harmful energies are being cleared from the target, situation, or location. The Increasing position shows that beneficial energies are being added or placed into the target, situation, or location.

L-Rods for Measuring Energy Fields

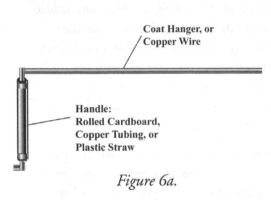

Coat Hanger, or
Copper Wire

Handle:
Rolled Cardboard,
Copper Tubing, or
Plastic Straw

Figure 6a.

An L-rod is a versatile tool by which you can locate and measure unseen energies and objects. It is also called an angle rod, swing rod, pointing rod, or dowsing rod. I find it the best instrument for measuring auric fields.

Make a homemade pair of L-rods from coat hangers, sturdy copper wire, or welding rod. The length of the top wire can be from 4 inches to more than 2 feet long. Usually it is 12 to 16 inches long. The handle can be a cardboard roll, copper or plastic tubing, or a simple plastic drinking straw. Or you can purchase copper L-rods at *www.divinerevelation.org*.

The Ready position for an L-rod is holding the handle loosely with the top wire straight ahead of

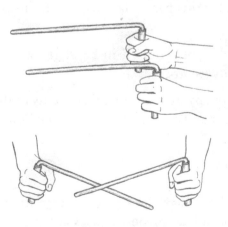

Figure 6b. Using L-rods

you, perpendicular to your body, with the tip of that wire tilting downward about 5 degrees. Do not clench the handle with a death-grip. You may place your thumb on top of the upper wire briefly to stop the wire from rotating. Then take your thumb off the wire; otherwise the rod will not swing freely. Keep your arms and hands comfortable and easy. If you tilt the tip of your rod too low, then gravity will take over and your rod will not swing. Keep the tilt at about 5 degrees.

One L-rod used alone can act as a pointer to find a lost object, hidden object, or direction. This is called Line of Bearing. The Ready position for one L-rod is straight ahead with tip slightly downward. The Found position for one rod is swinging sideways 90 degrees in one direction. One rod often indicates the Yes position by swinging to the right 90 degrees, and the No position by swinging left 90 degrees.

When two L-rods are used together, they are pointed forward for the Ready position. They usually cross for Yes position. For No position, they often swing outward, 180 degrees from each other. For Found position, the two L-rods may either cross or swing outward to indicate the target has been located.

L-Rod Positions

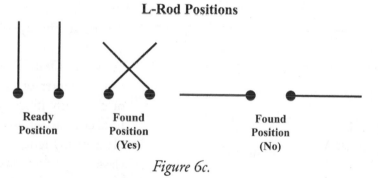

Ready
Position

Found
Position
(Yes)

Found
Position
(No)

Figure 6c.

Important: Before using your L-rods, do the Warm-Up Exercises described on page 236. You will then be in a relaxed, alert state of consciousness.

Hold your L-rod(s) easily and comfortably in Ready position. Now say out loud to your internal truth system, your higher self, or an aspect of the divine within (such as God, Holy Spirit, or another divine being), "Please show me the Yes position for my L-rod(s)."

Then take a few deep breaths and let go. Do what I call the "do-nothing program." That means do nothing, nothing, and less than nothing. Do not strain or have expectations. Do not try to elicit a response. Just take deep breaths and let go. Give up completely. Once you let go sufficiently, your L-rod(s) will swing into Yes position. If this position is different from what was described earlier, that is okay.

Then return your L-rod(s) to the Ready position. Tell your higher Self out loud, "Please show me the No position for my L-rod(s)." Make sure that your No position is readily distinguishable from your Yes position. Similarly, tell your higher self out loud, "Please show me the Found position for my L-rod(s)."

Then ask your higher self some questions to which you know the correct answer, such as, "Is my name _____?" Test to make sure your L-rod responds properly to the questions that you ask.

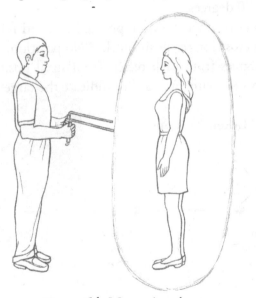

Figure 6d. Measuring Auras

If your L-rods do not respond, then you might consider hands-on training at a dowsing club meeting or conference. Go to *www.dowsers.org* and look for a local chapter or conference of the American Society of Dowsers or *www.ozarkresearch.org* for an Ozark Research Institute chapter or conference, or check my itinerary for my next class in Intuitive Kinesiology or my retreats or online classes at *www.susanshumsky.com.*

Duck-Beak Experiment

Now that you know how to use the L-rods, you can perform an interesting experiment with a friend. First, do the Warm-Up Exercises on page 236.

Ask your friend to stand on the other side of the room, facing you. Hold your two L-rods in Ready position. Say in a clear voice out loud, "Higher self [or God, or Holy Spirit, or Jesus, or another divine being], please show me the outer edge of [name of friend]'s blissful sheath." (See page 56 for more about the auric sheaths.)

Now, as you continue to point your L-rods at your friend, walk slowly toward your friend while remaining alert yet meditative, centered, balanced, and neutral. Do the "do-nothing program" as you walk. At some point, your L-rods will move into the Found position. That is the outer edge of your friend's blissful sheath.

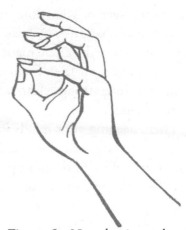

Figure 6e. Non-dominant hand

Now put aside your L-rods and do the following Duck-Beak Experiment along with your friend. With your non-dominant hand, create a circle between your pinky finger and your thumb. In other words, if you are right-handed, connect your left thumb tip with left pinky fingertip; if you are left-handed, connect your right pinky tip with right thumb tip. This will create a kind of electrical circuit.

Check your hand and make sure you have used your thumb and little (pinky) finger rather than your thumb and index (pointing) finger.

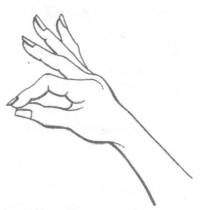

Figure 6f. Dominant hand

Then, with your dominant hand, make a little "duck" by pressing your thumb pad to your index finger pad. If you are right-handed, connect your right thumb to your right finger pad. Your three other fingers will be free, as though you are creating the shape of a duck-beak or a turkey with feathers.

Now stick the duck-beak into the hole. In other words, place your thumb

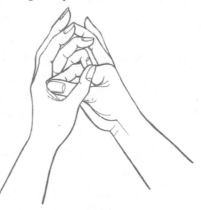

Figure 6g. Muscle-Testing

and index finger of your dominant hand into the circle made with your non-dominant hand. Your "beak" should stick up into your non-dominant palm from below the circle made by your non-dominant hand.

As you and your friend remain in this position, both say the following affirmation in a strong, clear, audible voice: "I AM a mighty, powerful, spiritual being."

Then, keeping your hands in the same position, try to pull apart the circle by opening your duck-beak. As your duck tries to open its mouth, press your pinky and thumb tips together and resist pressure, while applying an equal degree of pressure with your duck-beak. Press the duck-beak against the circle with steady continuous pressure, not a pumping action, and not forcing. As you resist the pressure with your non-dominant hand, you will find it difficult to open the circle with your duck-beak. This is called *muscle-testing* or *muscle-checking*.

Now pick up your L-rods and measure the outer edge of your friend's blissful sheath again. You may find that, after your friend has spoken this positive affirmation, his/her aura has grown larger.

Put your rods aside and both you and your friend assume the duck-beak hand position again. Remain in this position in a relaxed fashion, without pressing or resisting. Say the following affirmation audibly and clearly with your friend, as though you both really meant it: "I AM unworthy, inadequate, useless, and shameful."

Then muscle-test again by pressing your dominant hand's duck-beak against your non-dominant hand's circle, while you resist with equal pressure. You will find your circle will open easily, as scissors do, under the pressure applied by your duck-beak.

Now pick up your L-rods and measure the outer edge of your friend's blissful sheath again. You will likely find your friend's aura has shrunk significantly. It may only extend 12 inches or less from his/her body.

Put your L-rods aside and assume the duck-beak hand position again. Return to a relaxed attitude and both you and your friend say the following affirmation audibly in a strong, clear voice: "I AM divinely protected by the light of my being." Once more, when you practice muscle-testing, your circle will have strong resistance to your duck-beak. It will not open.

Pick up your L-rods and measure your friend's energy field again. You will find the aura has now expanded dramatically.

What did you learn from doing this amazing experiment? You might draw several conclusions:

 * Positive affirmations and truth statements strengthen your muscles. Negative affirmations and false statements weaken your muscles.

 * Positive affirmations and truth statements strengthen, energize, and expand your energy field dramatically. Negative affirmations and false statements weaken, deplete, and shrink your energy field dramatically.

 * The effects of positive and negative affirmations and statements demonstrate results immediately.

More Interesting Experiments

Here are some other experiments you might do with your friend:

 * Send positive thoughts, then negative thoughts, and then positive thoughts to your friend. Do not tell your friend which type of thought you are sending. Measure the aura and see the result.

 * Ask your friend to think positive, then negative, and then positive thoughts, without telling you which kind of thought he or she is thinking. Measure the aura after each type of thought.

 * Measure your friend's aura. Then tell the aura to stay there and ask your friend to go somewhere else. Measure the aura. It will no longer be around your friend. Then call the aura back to your friend and measure it again.

Using Muscle-Testing

Like L-rods, muscle-testing is a method that has a Yes, No, and Ready position. The Ready position for this method is pictured in Figure 6g on page 103. The Yes position is usually a strong circle with your non-dominant hand that cannot be opened by your dominant hand's duck-beak. The No position is a weak circle, which can easily be opened by your duck-beak.

Now test this for yourself by placing your hands in the muscle-testing Ready position. Then tell your higher self, "Please show me the Yes position for muscle-testing," and resist with your non-dominant hand while

Pendulum for Measuring Energy Fields

you attempt to open the circle with your duck-beak. Then repeat the process as you as ask for a No response.

How to Use a Pendulum

A pendulum is any kind of string, chain, or other armature attached to a weight. This can be a teabag on a string, a button or washer on a string, a curtain pull-cord, or a key, locket, or pocket watch on a chain. It can also be a pendulum created and designed for dowsing. Make your own pendulum or order one at *www .divinerevelation.org*.

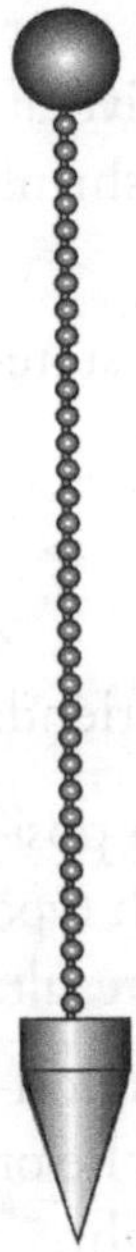

Like any other dowsing tool, a pendulum has a Ready, Yes, No, and Found position. Ask your higher self to show you these positions. Or program your pendulum to use the positions in Figure 6i. The Ready position is swinging at a 45-degree angle, as shown in the chart. The Yes position is swinging straight ahead forward and backward at a 90-degree angle, and the No position is swinging left and right, at a 180-degree angle.

Do the Warm-Up Exercises on page 236. Hold the string or chain of your pendulum between your thumb and index finger at any part of chain that is comfortable, leaving about 3 to 5 inches of it hanging. The chain's length will determine how fast it swings. As you shorten the armature or chain, the pendulum moves faster.

Hold the pendulum above the chart in Figure 6i. Then manually move the pendulum. Make it swing back and forth at a 45-degree angle, in Ready position. Continue to make it move. If necessary, tell your pendulum out loud to continue to swing in Ready position. The only part of the pendulum's swing that matters is the forward half of the swing. Ignore the backward swing (the dotted line on the chart).

Once your pendulum is swinging in Ready position, tell your higher self, "Please show me the Yes position for the pendulum." Take a few deep breaths and do the "do-nothing program." Your pendulum will continue swinging while gradually moving from Ready position toward the left, until it is moving straight forward and backward in Yes position on the chart.

Figure 6h.

Move your pendulum to the Ready position again, and ask for a No response. Your pendulum will move to the left again, from Ready position all the way to No position. Pay attention only to the forward half the swing, the half of the swing that is further away from you.

You might find your pendulum spins in circles, perhaps clockwise for a Yes response and counterclockwise for a No response. This is acceptable. However, it may limit you when using elaborate charts for detailed queries.

Finally, tell your higher self, "Please show me the Found position for the pendulum." Your Found position may be a circular movement or a backward-and-forward Yes position.

Pendulum Question Chart

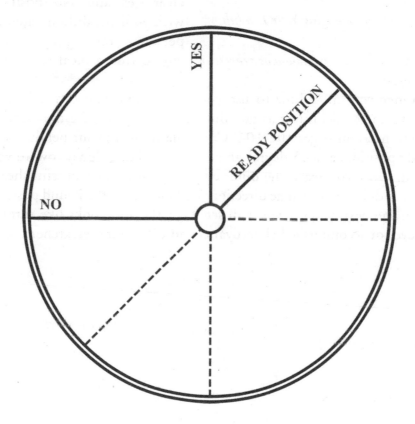

Figure 6i.

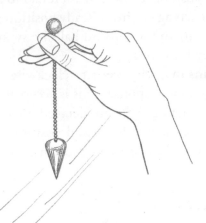

Figure 6j. Swinging Your Pendulum

In addition to this instruction, it is strongly recommended that you read and use *Letter to Robin—A Mini-Course in Pendulum Dowsing*, by Walt Woods. You can download this free e-book from *www .lettertorobin.org*.

After reading and using *Letter to Robin* to program your pendulum, if you still have trouble accomplishing clear Yes and No positions with your pendulum, then get personal training by visiting *www.dowsers.org* or *www.ozarkresearch.org* to find a local chapter or conference.

Once you know how to use your pendulum, you can measure a friend's energy field, just as you did with the L-rod. Use the same instructions as on pages 102-104. Continually swing your pendulum in Ready position, at a 45-degree angle, while walking slowly toward your friend. Once you reach the outer edge of your friend's blissful sheath, your pendulum will change directions and move into the Found position.

In the next chapter, you will see what the aura looks like through the eyes of accomplished clairvoyants and other aura researchers.

7

What Does Your Aura Look Like?

ଚ୍ଚ

Seeing Auras and Thought-Forms

"Dwelling in the light, there is no occasion at all for stumbling, for all things are discovered in the light."

—George Fox[1]

Your energy field is a veritable kaleidoscope of vibrant, shimmering hues, ever-shifting and colliding with your moods and thoughts. These colors are the outer display of continually changing inner vibratory states underlying your emotions. Patches of color, streaks, stripes, dots, flashes, streams, or clouds may appear and disappear. Black clouds may obscure the bright color beneath.

When you are feeling particularly serene, your aura may appear calm, luminous, and radiant, like a halo. When you are emotionally upset or excited, it might blaze as a fiery furnace, burning building, or explosion, with flames shooting out, dancing,

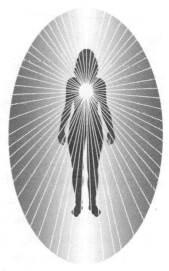

Figure 7a. Radiant Aura

109

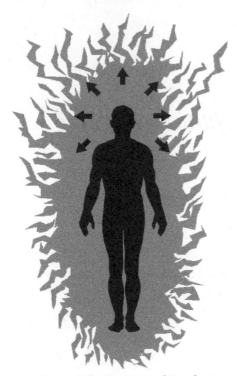

Figure 7b. Emotional Explosion

or swirling in a chaotic maelstrom. These flames might detach from your aura and dart into the atmosphere.

Your aura is never completely at rest. Even during relaxation, mental calm, or meditation, a pulsing, wavelike motion vibrates throughout your aura. When your emotions are at a crescendo, nearly anyone can feel the intense, wild vibrational storms spewing from your energy field, even without seeing the colors.

Auric Research Studies

Since the beginning of the 20th century, research into the human energy field led to observations of a luminous glow around living organisms. Here are findings of some pioneers in this field.

Kilner: Auric Field

In 1911 Walter J. Kilner, MD (1847–1920), of St. Thomas Hospital in London, published extensive studies of the human aura. Looking through glass screens stained with dicyanin dye called *spectauranine*, he observed multicolored, oval haloes with three distinct zones, with the densest portion closest to the body.

Kilner found that male auras are alike, independent of age, yet the auras of girls differ from those of women. Male auras are larger at the head and then follow the body's contours. Female child auras are similar to males', but adult female auras are wider than males', especially at the waist (extending 6 to 12 inches from the body). When women stand sideways, their auras are widest at the small of the back, chest, and abdomen.

Kilner's observations could explain why men are stereotypically categorized as rational and head-centered, whereas women are considered emotional and heart-centered.

Kilner found that fatigue, disease, mood, hypnosis, magnetism, and electricity all alter aura size and color. He diagnosed and treated major diseases based on the aura's color, structure, volume, and presence. Kilner's work, which was greeted with skepticism by the medical profession, was interrupted by the onset of World War I.

Pierrakos: Bioenergetics

John C. Pierrakos, MD (1921–2001), Greek-born psychiatrist, scientist, cofounder of Institute for Bioenergetic Analysis in New York, cofounder of Core Energetics, and codirector of The Energy Research Group, studied energy fields of humans, animals, plants, and crystals for 12 years with his colleague, Alexander Lowen.

Pierrakos portrayed the energy field as "a light cast of the body energies," and he defined energy as "the living force emanated by consciousness." He said that humans "swim in a sea of fluid, tinged rhythmically with brilliant colors which constantly change hues, shimmer, and vibrate. For being alive is to be colorful and vibrant."[2]

Pierrakos reported three layers of the field:

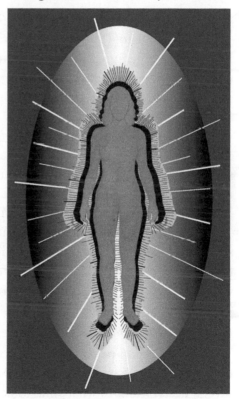

1. Inner layer: one-fifth to one-eight inch thick; dark blue-black, violet, or ultraviolet; empty, transparent, and crystalline.

2. Middle layer: 3 to 4 inches thick; blue-gray in color; brilliant, shimmering, liquid, and rarified, displaying:

   a. A wavelike form filling the entire layer.

Figure 7c. Aura Layers

b. An overall *Brownian motion* appearance (that is, like masses of
particles suspended in liquid, moving randomly).
c. White or yellow rays projecting several feet from the body with
a fringed effect around the head.
3. Outer layer: 6 to 8 inches thick; nearly transparent sky-blue;
expanding up to 100 feet, with spiral or vortical movement
and diffused, indistinct boundaries.

Pierrakos found the energy field is affected by activity, rest, metabolism, emotions, and breathing rate and quality. Its motion is continuous, complex, ever-changing, pulsating, and vibrating. Streams of energy radiate toward the head and feet simultaneously. Vibrations extend past the body's boundaries. By studying these characteristics, pathological conditions can be determined.

Hunt: Biofield and Aura Color

From 1970 to 1990 Dr. Valerie Hunt, head of UCLA's Physiology Department, measured the human biofield during Rolfing sessions. Electrodes on subjects' skin recorded low millivoltage signals, while clairvoyant aura readers Rosalyn Bruyere and Barbara Brennan observed their auras.

Scientists then mathematically evaluated the wave patterns by Fourier analysis and sonogram frequency analysis, which exactly correlated with specific colors. In other words, where readers saw blue, electronic measurements showed the characteristic blue waveform and frequency. In 1988 Hunt successfully repeated this experiment with seven other aura readers: "Throughout the centuries in which sensitives [those who can perceive subtle energies] have seen and described the auric emissions, this is the first objective electronic evidence of frequency, amplitude and time, which validates their subjective observation of color discharge."[3]

What Aura Readers See

Depending on personal experience, mental ideas, biases, and so forth, clairvoyants differ widely in their aura interpretations. In this chapter are several descriptions of what auras look like. However, I suggest you do your own research in viewing the auric field.

Good aura readers can distinguish two unique layers of your energy field. The first is an underlying, semi-permanent color determined by character, awareness, and habits. The second layer is shaped by temporary moods and thought-forms (congealed energy built of habits and beliefs), in continual flux.

Although your aura surrounds your entire body, the densest portion is around your head and shoulders. Intense colors usually indicate greater willpower, focused energy, spirit, and vivacity. Many factors contribute to aura appearance, including food, health, and environment. But the most important factor is mind.

Auras of pregnant and nursing women exhibit bright, easily visible auras of soft, pastel colors. Public speakers, singers, and musicians display brilliant, colorful auras when they perform with emotion and enthusiasm. Children's auras often appear smaller than adults, but what is lacking in size is more than compensated by color strength, brightness, and vibrancy, and significantly greater open chakras than in adults.

Drug addicts, alcoholics, and mentally ill individuals exhibit gray clouds of astral mucous. Astral entities often display black or gray spheres. In contrast, spiritual guides, angels, divine teachers, and departed loved ones emit brilliant white balls of energy, frequently appearing near the head. Tiny orbs are often deceased pets. New babies emerge as small balls of light to the right of the mother-to-be.

According to Barbara Brennan, author of *Hands of Light*, auras of particularly defensive individuals are enveloped by a hard, thick shell that prevents intimacy (Figure 7d). A person making excuses or verbally denying accusations displays a large halo projecting around the head (Figure 7e). Someone with a superior attitude exhibits a bulging aura

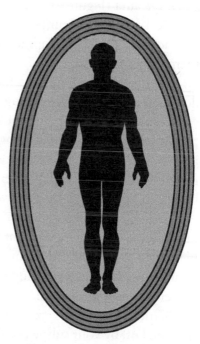

Figure 7d. Defensiveness

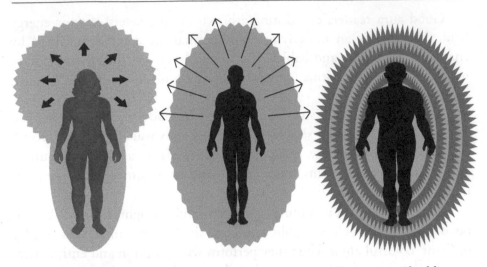

Figure 7e. Verbal Denial   Figure 7f. Superiority   Figure 7g. Shielding

projecting in all directions, which is called a *puffed-up*, *swelled-head*, or *inflated-ego* aura (Figure 7f). A shrunken or collapsed aura surrounds people who feel inferior, incompetent, unworthy, or undeserving. Deeply hurt individuals build a porcupine-like shield, preventing others getting near them (Figure 7g).

During waking hours, colorful emotional-body thought-forms predominate the aura. But during sleep, when mind and body are resting, your astral-vital body is foremost. Then, your aura becomes a semitransparent pearly or milky field, tinged with opalescent hues and tints, blending, shifting, hiding, and reappearing. This radiant pearly substance is your *etheric double*, or *vital body*, an exact replica of your human body. This vital body can shrink or expand, however.

Your aura is filled with infinitesimal sparkling energy particles resembling electric sparks in constant motion. This vibratory movement resembles steam or heat rising from your body. Because the pranic particles in your energy field are breathing life into your body, this dancing movement is literally the dance of life.

With every breath you exhale, minute subtle energy particles are sloughed off by your subtle body. These particles remain in the atmosphere for a long time and leave a scent detectable by dogs, cats, and other animals.

What Are Thought-Forms?

Have you ever felt someone become upset? Did you ever see anger in someone's eyes? Have you ever sensed a person's feelings? Perhaps anxious, sad, guilty, scary, or weird feelings? Upon first meeting someone, did you notice arrogance, timidity, confidence, shyness, cruelty, fear, or discomfort? If you answered yes to any of these questions, then you have seen or felt thought-forms.

Thought-forms are strong emotions, feelings, ideas, habits, patterns, or conditioning energized by powerful willpower. Corresponding intense vibrations create powerful energy vortices of thought-force in a field of strongly cohesive auric substance, charged with pranic energy. Pranic material forms the building blocks of thought-forms, which display vibrant colors and energies.

Some thought-forms are semi-permanent, such as those comprising your mental body. Others are temporary and fade in and out with moods. Some thought-forms, called *façade bodies* or *rakshasas*, appear to have a life of their own, taking on a unique, almost independent personality (see pages 184 and 188).

Your thought-forms can exert a powerful influence. They can become so imbued with pranic energy and mental willpower that they flare projectiles of lightning into the atmosphere. Anyone in the path of these flashes of thought will feel the brunt of tangible energy in a visceral way.

Thought-forms are energetic beings created by your mind, will, and pranic substance. They are children of your mind, birthed of thought substance and life essence. They may live for a few seconds, or they may persist as semi-permanent fixtures of your mental body or even establish themselves as separate entities outside your aura. As heat remains in a room after a fireplace has died out, thought-forms sometimes remain after the person who created them has left the premises.

What Do Thought-Forms Look Like?

Thought-forms often appear in your aura as undulating waves, similar to the surface of a lake. Others look like whirling, cloudy energy balls, vortices, whirlpools, or pinwheels. Some emerge as smoke spiraling from a locomotive or a diesel truck. Great jets might spew the way steam spurts from a teakettle, or spout in one jet or a series of jets. Thought-forms may resemble powerful beams of lightning, flashes of soft light, or corkscrews boring into space. Immeasurably beautiful geometric forms or patterns may glow with phosphorescent light.

Thought-forms usually display simple colors, because the emotion underlying them is one-dimensional. For example, thought-forms of intense anger often appear as characteristic red and black flashes or streaks of lightning. People often say "my temper flared"—and, quite literally, it did. Passion might manifest as dark red. A thought-form of unconditional love may manifest as a flower with beautiful pink petals.

The appearance of thought-forms can be influenced by other people. In the 1960s, Thelma Moss researched the human energy field with her high-voltage camera in the UCLA radiation field photography lab. In one study, pairs of individuals held their fingertips close together without touching as they stared into each other's eyes. Frequently, for no apparent explanation, one of the fingertips would practically disappear. Later it was discovered that one subject was a professional hypnotist who could blank out the fingertip of a number of his partners.

In another striking experiment, one subject imagined sticking a needle into her partner, who was afraid of needles. The high-voltage photograph showed a sharp red line darting out of the aggressor's finger toward her imagined victim, whose corona appeared to recoil. In another case, a photograph of two individuals taken while meditating together showed a merging of their two individual coronas.

Thought-forms can stay in your energy field or travel enormous distances. Some fade out as they travel. Others continue to faintly glow in the atmosphere for a long time. Space is no barrier to projecting thought-forms. They can travel anywhere.

The most emotionally charged thought-forms take the shape of bombs that figuratively explode when they reach their target. Often, intense thought-bombs are projected to an audience by public speakers, orators, or politicians.

Some extreme thought-forms literally push people back or attack their targets with mental arrows, which can displace the auric field. Others coil around or tie a person in a knot. Still others lasso and drag the target aura toward its instigator. Such phenomena are accompanied by intense emotional coercion and intimidation. An octopus thought-form with long, winding, clinging tentacles may attack the solar plexus or wrap around and suffocate the target. Such psychic manipulation, caused by emotional neediness, tends to draw the aura down or grapple it toward the perpetrator.

Life-enhancing or life-damaging thought-forms project positive or negative vibrations, depending on the instigator. In one case, a beauteous, rainbow-colored light-shaft streamed downward over a man's left shoulder while he received inspiration from his higher self as he wrote, lectured, and taught in an effort to help and lift others.

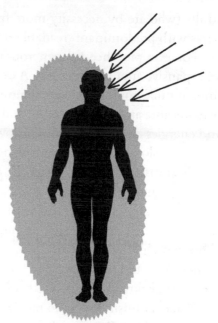

Figure 7h. Mental Arrow Attack

Your aura is a self-charging field that never runs out of energy as long as your body remains alive. In contrast, thought-forms, with no internal power source, are temporary. They live only as long as the battery power of the initial energy thrust that created them will allow.

Auric Personalities

Auras can often give insights into the character or personality of a person. Habits, thoughts, and diseases are revealed by the shape and coloration of thought-forms. The aura of an ordinary individual radiates about two feet from the body.

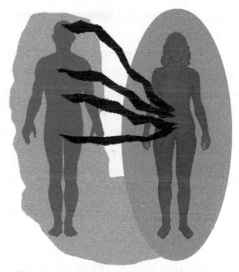

Figure 7i. Octopus Thought-Form

Its coloration varies from clear and radiant to dark and murky, depending on emotions and health. Whereas children's auras are in continual flux, adults (who are by necessity more fixed in their ways) display more stable auras with predominant, readable traits.

For example, cheerful, generous individuals are frequently imbued with an expansive aura of soft colors. A loving, big-hearted nature appears as soft tints of pink, rose, light blue, lemon, and pale green. In contrast, a greedy person's aura appears contracted and small, with dirty brown-orange colors and energies channeled into a narrow focus. Circulation is curtailed. There is neither sloughing off of toxins nor input from universal energies. The aura is encased in an impenetrable, confining crust of small boundaries of loneliness and helplessness.

A sensual person obsessed with carnal pleasure often shows a crimson, scarlet, and deep, dirty blue or muddy purple energy field. If he or she conceives children, the aura gradually changes with the development of familial love and devotion. The focus of vibrations shifts from the sacral to the heart chakra. The harsh red colors transform into rose and blue.

Practical businesspeople motivated by material pursuits often display an orange aura. Because their intellects dominate their hearts, the aura around their head is large and prominent.

A shy individual may display weak colors or a color void on the right side of the body. Conversely, an extrovert may have a deficient aura on the left side.

A spiritual person's aura is often blue or violet with light blue, green, and violet radiating from the heart. Such a glorious auric field is seen in humble, often illiterate people who sacrifice for others: nursing the sick, helping the poor, uplifting the aged.

Educators who serve humanity display auras with both head and heart centers vibrating powerful energies. These individuals exhibit an exalted, glowing yellow, white, lemon, or blue color. In the heart center, such lovers of humanity radiate devotional colors of mauve, purple, or blue.

A true saint, or *mahatma* ("great soul"), exhibits a large, shining, fluorescent, pearly white auric field, spanning several feet around the body. In such enlightened individuals, radiation from the thousand-petaled lotus above the head imbues the entire auric field with incandescent, silvery, shimmering luminosity. Anyone sensitive to vibrations can feel the warm glow of such a powerfully loving aura.

How to Read the Health of the Aura

When life force is flowing powerfully through the energy field, aura colors are bright, vibrant, and pulsating. In most people, the energy field is largest above the waist. In the healthiest individuals, the aura is the same size all around the body.

Your vital sheath, or pranic aura, is nearly colorless—the color of clear water or a perfect diamond. In a particularly healthy, vibrant individual, it glows with a faint, warm pink tinge. Clairvoyants perceive it as streaked or marked by minute, bristle-like lines radiating outward. In healthy auras, the bristle-like streaks appear stiff and brittle. When health is deficient, the radiations look tangled, mangled, twisted, curly, or drooping.

Illness often appears as a collapsed, squished aura or area of darkness. Some aura readers call this a *hole* or *energy leak*. Dark holes often appear in the energy field over an area of illness.

For example, with lung cancer, the dark spot would appear in the front and/or back of the aura, right over the tumor.

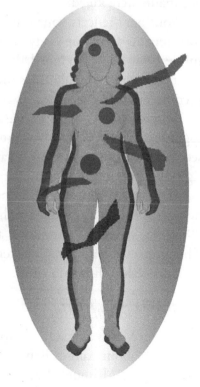

The remarkable psychic Edgar Cayce (1877–1945) once knew a man who always wore blue, even down to his tie and socks. One day this "blue man" went to the store and surprised himself by buying several maroon ties. Then he bought shirts with garnet stripes and scarlet ties and handkerchiefs. He continued to wear red clothing for several years. Meanwhile his health deteriorated. He became increasingly nervous and tired. Eventually he had a nervous breakdown.

During this time the color red grew in his auric field. Then gray, the color of illness, crept into the red. But as he recuperated, blue began to eat up the red. Eventually blue won the battle and the man recovered. He never wore red again.[4]

Figure 7j. Energy leaks

Another friend of Cayce was a woman who saw colorful auras during childhood. She thought everyone did. One day this child met a woman whom the child thought was peculiar, though she could not pinpoint why. When the child got home, it struck her that the woman had no colors around her. Within a few weeks the woman was dead.[5]

Edgar Cayce was always able to see auras. One day he was waiting for an elevator on the sixth floor of a department store. As he waited, some bright red sweaters attracted his attention. Then the elevator arrived, full of people, and he stepped forward to enter it. However, something stopped Cayce dead in his tracks. Though the car was well lit, it appeared dark to Cayce. He was repelled by this energy and told the elevator operator to go ahead. As he stepped over to the red sweaters, Cayce realized what had made him uneasy: The people in the elevator had no auras. At that moment, the elevator cable snapped, the car fell to the basement, and all its occupants were killed.

Your aura reflects your soul's vibrations. When death draws near, the soul retreats from the body. There is no color in the aura, because the subtle body has abandoned the physical body and is hovering above it. Then the aura gradually fades until the withdrawal from the earthly form is complete.

Surprisingly, you can see auras around people on television or in photographs. Because people who are near death or dead have no aura, a corpse seen on a newscast will show no aura. Photographs or films of people taken right before death display no aura.

If a plane is about to crash, passengers boarding that plane will exhibit no auric field. When the space shuttle Challenger was boarded on January 29, 1986, the seven astronauts' auras no longer surrounded their bodies. Therefore, the photograph taken just before the crewmembers boarded their spaceship shows no auras.

Seeing Celestial Beings

Kathy Martin, an aura photographer from Santa Fe, Texas, had always wondered about balls of light she observed around people's heads in their aura photos. Although Kathy was told these light spheres were divine inner teachers, deities, angelic beings, and other divine beings, she did not believe it. She was looking for a face and wings. So she decided to pray for a definitive answer.

Soon afterward, Kathy was taking aura photos in New York City. As she waited for an aura photo to develop, the woman whose photo she had just taken said, "I can see guardian angels and loved ones, and they appear as balls of light around the shoulder area. Sometimes they are so bright that I ask them to tone down their light so I can concentrate on the person I am talking to."

By that time the aura photo had developed. Kathy peeled off the backing. When the woman saw the photograph, she screamed, "That's it! That's what I see!" Just then, thousands of goose bumps and rushes of energy ran through

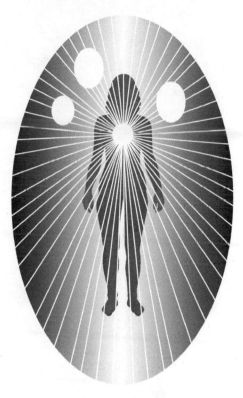

Figure 7k. Divine Beings

Kathy's body. A divine voice came to Kathy clearly: "We are not a physical body. Quit looking for one. We are light."

As you observe auras, remember that you are looking through your own auric field. Therefore, your own thought-forms and emotions may color your observations. Because studying auras is a new field of research, you can become a pioneer in the field.

In the next chapter, you will learn how to interpret colors that you observe in the human energy field.

8

What Color Is Your Aura?

ﬠﬠ

Discovering Light and Color

"You must not think of the light of the sun as the true Light of God. It is a reflection of the true Light."

—Omraam M. Aivanhov[1]

Probably the first thing that comes to mind when you hear the word *aura* is color. That is because we imagine that aura readers look at colors in our energy field and then interpret their meanings. With this in mind, in this chapter we will see how color relates to the human energy field.

Many children naturally see light around people. The invariable rebuff from the majority of parents is "You are just imagining it." As a child, a clairvoyant named Maretha told her mother that a neighbor's "light was going out." Her mother became extremely upset when the neighbor suddenly died. She scolded Maretha, "Never talk like that again."[2]

Joseph's "coat of many colors" in the Bible is an ancient allusion to a great prophet's auric raiment (meaning "radiant"), indicating his high degree of spiritual attainment. Joseph's envious brothers stole this precious coat, cast him into a pit, and sold him into slavery for 20 pieces of silver. Yet Joseph accurately interpreted Pharaoh's dream and saved the entire kingdom from starvation. He was honored as ruler over all of Egypt.[3]

Aura Color Meanings

Light is life. This is the first manifestation of creation: "Let there be light: and there was light."[4] The sun's white light is a mere reflection of the pure light of the Holy Spirit, perceived only by the inner eye. This divine light manifests in your aura as seven cosmic "rays" of pranic energy. Although all seven rays appear in your energy field, the underlying color indicates which cosmic ray you are most aligned with.

It is said in the Bible, "Thou shalt love the Lord thy God with all thy heart, and with all thy soul, and with all thy strength, and with all thy mind; and thy neighbour as thyself."[5] Loving God with your heart fulfills the green ray. Loving God with your mind fulfills the yellow ray; with your soul, fulfills the indigo and violet rays; and with your strength, fulfills the orange and red rays. When you love God and your neighbor completely, you unify with the white light of Spirit, which encompasses all rays.

Pure white light is a mixture of all colors of the rainbow. Black is the absence of color. The longest visible wavelength is red, and the shortest is violet.

Electromagnetic Radiations

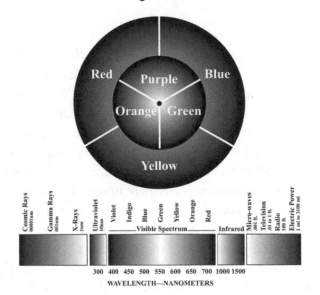

Figure 8a.

Radiant and Reflected Light

Color rays are transmitted in two ways:

1. Through radiant light sources.
2. Reflected from surfaces.

Color coming from the sun, a projector, a computer screen, or a television screen is radiant light. Color on paper, clothing, walls, furniture, or paintings is reflected light.

The primary colors of radiant light differ from primary colors of reflected light. Radiant light primary colors are red, green, and purple. When these three are mixed, pure white light results. When red and green light are mixed, yellow light appears. Purple and red light generate mauve, and green and purple make blue. Radiant colors mixed together are brighter and more potent than the original colors.

In contrast, reflected pigments have different primary colors: red, yellow, and blue. Mixing these three pigments produces white. Reflected colors are specific wavelengths reflecting from a surface. When all light reflects from a surface, white appears. When all light is absorbed, black results. Violet cloth absorbs all color rays of white light except violet. With no light source, any surface appears black.

Through mixing the primary pigments of red, yellow, and blue, secondary colors are created: red and yellow make orange; yellow and blue create green; red and blue produce violet. By continuing to mix colors, all possible colors result. Mixing colors directly opposite each other on the color wheel (called *complimentary colors*) results in gray. (See Figure 8b on page 126.) Adding white makes any color lighter and is called a *tint*. Adding black makes it darker, in which case it is a *shade*.

Unlike radiant light, when two reflected pigments are mixed, less light reflects in the resulting pigment. Therefore, no pigments can match the brilliance of nature's colors or sunlight.

Auric light is neither radiant (from the sun) nor reflected (from a surface). Its light is more potent than either—it is cosmic spiritual light. However, in aura interpretation, primary colors are red, yellow, and blue. There are no "bad" or "good" colors. Every color has value, because particular physical, mental, or emotional states exhibit different colors at different times. Therefore, rushing to judgment when reading auras is unwise.

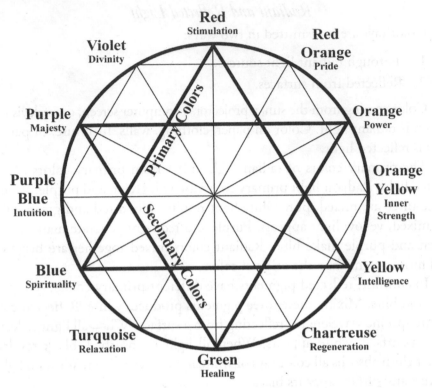

Figure 8b. Color Wheel

Red

In ancient symbolism red is the color of the physical human body, the earth, and hell. All physical activity, whether vitalizing or depleting, manifests red vibrations.

Yellow

The ancient meaning of the color yellow is the mind. All intellectual activity, whether uplifting or degrading, demonstrates yellow vibrations.

Blue

Blue is the color of heaven and Spirit in ancient symbolism. All forms of religious feeling, whether truly spiritual or fanatical, exhibit blue vibrations.

White

White stands for pure Spirit, the essence of all that is, the most positive quality in the universe.

Black

Black is the color of negation, the absence of light. It is the negative polarity, the opposite of the white vibration.

> WHITE = Positivism—Infinite Light
> BLUE = Spirit—Spiritual
> YELLOW = Mind—Intellectual
> RED = Body—Physical
> BLACK = Negation—Infinite Darkness

Because cosmic rays are pure, unmixed colors, auras with bright, clear colors reflect a positive, healthy attitude and energy. By mixing colors, the entire spectrum of mental and emotional activities is represented. For example, yellow and blue create green—a mixture of intellect and spirituality. Adding white brightens the aura. Adding black or a complimentary color results in dark, murky colors, signifying toxic emotions or illness. In this case, the flow of divine energy is impeded, like a pure beam of sunlight filtered through a dirty window, blocking much of the light. In this book you will learn profound ways to keep your energy field clear, pristine, and bright.

Red Ray—Vitality

The red cosmic ray carries pure life-force. In the scriptures of India, the energy of prana is described as being red in color. Pure red is the color of healthy blood as it leaves the heart, filled with oxygen. A ruddy complexion denotes health. In contrast, skin pallor implies illness. Thus red in the aura represents health, strength, vigor, and virility. Strong, healthy children often exhibit a pure red aura.

Red predominating an adult aura may indicate materialism and physical needs. Red denotes the deepest passions, whether love or hatred. Righteous indignation emits brilliant, pure, scarlet flames. Vibrant crimson represents pure love. Rose red means love of family and country. Light red signifies nervousness and impulsiveness. Scarlet indicates egotism.

Dark red indicates domineering tendencies. Unmitigated lust, motivated by self-indulgent greed, emanates blackish red. Muddy red leaping flames against a black background represent malicious hatred. Similar flames against green symbolize jealousy or envy. Avarice is a combination of dull, dark red and dirty, muddy green.

- ⚶ **Bright red:** enthusiasm, vitality, strength, determination, perseverance, seeking perfection, strong will, leadership, courage, spirit, animation, movement, love, warmth, friendship, affection, generosity, sacrifice, sensitivity to others, humility, self-knowledge, introspection, healthy ambition, physical exercise, companionship, healthy sports.

- ⚶ **Dark red:** self-preservation, selfishness, hurriedness, impulsiveness, infantile tendencies, selfish affection, high temper, nervousness, turmoil, turbulence, control, domination.

- ⚶ **Muddy red:** anger, hatred, frustration, greed, cruelty, rage, reactivity, defiance, vengeance, violence, destruction, aggression, domination, hostile competition, sensuality, unbridled sexual lust, blood lust.

Pink Ray—Love

A high vibration of unselfish, spiritual, devotional, universal love manifests a beautiful rose-tinted aura. Pink is perfect balance between spiritual (purple) and material (red) life. The most advanced souls display a rare, large pink aura. The term "rose-colored glasses" refers to optimism, uplift, inspiration, motivation, and cheerfulness, and "in the pink" indicates health.

Coral (orange-pink) represents immaturity and is often seen in children. In adults it indicates delayed adolescence, childish selfishness, fear of making choices, or unhappiness with the environment.

- ⚶ **Bright pink:** unconditional love, kindness, openness, compassion, sympathy, empathy, charity, generosity, modesty, refinement, artistic nature, cheerfulness, health, joy, comfort, companionship, increased activity.

ॐ **Muddy pink:** lustful passion, childish emotions, selfishness, critical, judgmental mind, lack of joy, conditional love, unkindness, defensiveness, insecurity.

Orange Ray–Power

In the early Christian church, orange was the color of glory, virtue, and fruits of the earth. This color indicates power—the ability or desire to inspire or control others. As combined yellow and red, orange implies mental vigor, intellectual ambition, pride, and mastery by willpower. Bright amber indicates inner strength and intellectual mastery.

Orange tinged with red suggests an overly domineering, controlling nature. Medium orange-red, a vitalizing color, emanates from the fingers of conscientious physicians. People first turning from materialism to intellectualism may display orange auras. Sometimes this color indicates kidney problems.

ॐ **Bright orange:** optimism, self-confidence, emotional balance, spontaneity, creativity, enthusiasm, motivation, ambition, inspiration, courage, leadership, tactfulness, self-mastery, self-control, intellectual mastery, willpower, thoughtfulness, consideration, discernment, hospitality, friendliness, cooperation, humanitarianism.

ॐ **Muddy orange:** indifference, laziness, apathy, emotional instability, fear of failure, lack of self-confidence, nervousness, repression, overbearing, forcefulness, coercion, manipulation, self-absorption, selfish pride, self-indulgence, superficiality, pretense, social climbing, power-seeking, insensitivity, suspicion, condemnation, criticism, being antisocial.

Gold Ray–Wisdom

Pure intellectual attainment and pure love of knowledge manifest a clear golden yellow aura. Powerful spiritual masters of great wisdom display a golden halo around their heads, tinged with a border of blue, and pink in the outer layer. Buddha, Jesus, Krishna, and other great saints are depicted with a golden halo. People with clear, golden yellow auras do not worry, love to learn, and learn with ease.

৪ **Bright gold:** wisdom, knowledge, inspiration, health, wellbeing, happiness, friendliness, helpfulness, mastery, attunement with God.

৪ **Muddy gold or tan:** fear, timidity, inferiority, indecisiveness, weak will, dependency, camouflage, hiding.

Yellow Ray—Intellect

Yellow denotes the mental realm devoid of any traces of earthly life. Therefore, clear, bright, radiant yellow auras appear in those with highest intellect, curiosity, adventure, optimism, and love of knowledge. Lemon yellow implies mental strength for artistic works or scientific inventions. Healers with light yellow auras can calm frazzled nerves and bring a quiet, balanced presence.

A reddish tinge indicates indecisiveness or inferiority complex. Very pale yellow indicates illness. Muddy or murky yellow denotes fear, timidity, or terror. Calling someone "yellow" implies cowardice.

৪ **Bright yellow:** joy, mental power, clear thinking, vision, logic, reason, patience, self-control, adventure, acceptance, intellectualism, inquisitiveness, optimism, happiness, friendliness, wisdom, helpfulness, creativity, precision, flexibility, efficiency, analysis, organization, problem-solving.

৪ **Muddy yellow:** fear, bitterness, greed, regret, fear of unknown, weak will, timidity, mental/verbal aggression, confusion, criticism, skepticism, overanalyzing, mental overstimulation, headache, judgment, egotism, isolation.

Green Ray—Harmony

Green is the color of healing and healers. In the early Christian church, this color represented youthfulness, fertility, and fields of springtime. In the very center of the spectrum, green balances two electromagnetic extremes. Thus, it signifies equilibrium and adaptability.

A pure, grass-green aura indicates a green thumb, love of nature, outdoor life, new beginnings, or tranquil home life. Light, pure green tints represent altruism and charity. A green aura, quivering as it rises through the energy field, indicates a most empathetic healer. A duller shade brings tact, diplomacy, and cooperation. Those with blue-green auras are trust-worthy and helpful. Turquoise auras indicate influential, organized, dynamic multitaskers.

A dull slate or olive color represents vile, depraved, tricky deceit and treachery. The murkiest green shows resentful malice—someone "green with envy" or a "green-eyed monster." Deceitful, lemony-green streaks often shoot just above people's heads when they are being evasive or lying.

- **Bright green:** healing, love, balance, harmony, peace, faith, hope, grace, attunement to divine will, brotherhood, cooperation, helpfulness, growth, change, loving service, mercy, learning, adaptability, higher awareness, tolerance, love of nature, friendliness, strength, prosperity.

- **Muddy green:** envy, jealousy, treachery, malice, apprehension, rigidity, inflexibility, stubbornness, selfishness, insecurity, self-doubt, miserliness, insincerity, shiftiness, deceit, treachery, mistrust, possessiveness.

Blue Ray–Spirituality

Blue is the color of Spirit, contemplation, prayer, and heaven, symbolizing religious, mystical, and spiritual feelings. In the early Christian church, blue was associated with highest attainments of the soul. Bright, clear, light sky-blue shows genuine spirituality. Pale blue shows less maturity but sincere desire to make efforts in the right direction. Aqua auras indicate harmony and balance. Such people work harder and more effectively than those with pale blue auras.

High morality, higher consciousness, deep spiritual understanding, and high ideals exhibit clear, brilliant sky-blue tints. "True blue" means sincerity in all relations. Deep, clear blue auras fulfill a mission toward unselfish ideals. Blue emanates from anyone set in the right direction toward a higher purpose, whether spiritual, artistic, or scientific. People with blue auras are born survivors—calm, relaxed, balanced, and quiet.

In contrast, bluish-gray indicates religious fundamentalism, overconscientiousness, timidity, or religion shadowed by fear and misgiving. Deep blue-black represents crude, superstitious beliefs. Heavy-heartedness or "feeling blue" appears as blackish or brownish-blue storm clouds.

     ᛦ   **Bright blue:** tranquility, composure, inspiration, intuition, spirituality, faith, devotion, self-reliance, loyalty, sensory introversion, caring, sensitivity, empathy, compassion, tolerance, wisdom, morality, honesty, selflessness, patience, gentleness, artistic creativity, contentment, following divine will, desire to experience God.

     ᛦ   **Muddy blue:** fear, procrastination, laziness, cool indifference, victimization, despondency, melancholy, self-pity, self-centeredness, stubbornness, struggle, rigidity, conservatism, suppressed feelings, fanaticism, intolerance, adherence to dogma, authoritarianism, self-righteousness, self-satisfaction, dependency on past.

Purple Ray–Intuition

Royal purple, the early color of kingly vestments, indicates high spiritual attainment, self-discipline, and dominion when displayed in the aura. The color of form, ritual, and solemn ceremony, purple is connected with religious titles and grandeur. This color was associated with humiliation and sorrow in the early Christian church.

Purple and violet represent all seekers—those searching for a cause or a spiritual experience. Purple successfully deals with practical, worldly matters. Blue-purple indicates accomplishment through divine power. Red-purple denotes human will and effort. Lavender indicates humility and worship.

     ᛦ   **Bright purple:** worldly or spiritual dominion, higher perception, intuition, ESP, divine wisdom, visionary abilities, self-discipline, hopeful expectations, idealistic ambitions.

     ᛦ   **Muddy purple:** fanaticism, religious fervor, possessiveness, overbearing, confusion, forgetfulness, inefficiency, preoccupation with future, introversion, nondiscipline, incompetence.

Violet Ray–Divine Realization

Violet, the highest frequency in the spectrum, represents the loftiest spiritual, religious feelings, thought, and attainment. Blue and red, combining aspiration and fortitude, blend in violet. Such an auric color indicates advanced consciousness.

The early Christian church used violet on penitential days to lift worshippers' thoughts from mundane concerns to heavenly harmony. Dreamy, visionary individuals with a high degree of spiritual, mental, and physical fortitude display violet auras. Because ultraviolet light destroys bacteria and parasites, healers with violet auras can assist the ill and distressed without catching contagious diseases. Heart or stomach trouble is often found in those with violet auras.

- **Bright violet:** divine realization, connection with God, unity consciousness, humility, creative imagination, vision, inspiration, freedom of spirit, high spiritual attunement, sensitivity to subtle energies, spiritual enlightenment.

- **Muddy violet:** fanaticism, religious fervor, possessiveness, absentmindedness, self-hatred, fantasy, nonconformity, unfaithfulness, unawareness of spirituality, ungroundedness, mental instability.

White Ray–Purity

If your soul were in perfect balance, then your entire auric spectrum would blend into a perfect, harmonious white color. White, the color of pure light and pure Spirit, raises the vibration of any color it mixes with. The white light of pure consciousness is radiant, pure energy, which transcends all light from the physical, mental, or spiritual planes. This aura color symbolizes a high degree of spiritual attainment and evolution. An individual with white permeating the entire auric field is a genuine spiritual master.

Pearly white indicates kindness, gentleness, and forgiveness. Oyster white means the soul is working hard to unfold higher awareness despite difficulties. Dirty white may indicate severe illness or drug abuse.

- **Bright white:** self-mastery, oneness with higher self, attunement with master, God realization.

- **Dirty white:** serious disease, often seen just before death, artificial stimulation from drugs, lack of mental and physical harmony.

Black—Withdrawal

The color black in the energy field is the absence of light, yet it brings light into higher focus. The darker the night sky, the more brilliantly the luminous stars and moon shine. Therefore black is not inherently "evil." At night all creatures on this planet rest and recuperate. Thus black, the color of sleep, suggests rejuvenation. Sleep indicates absence of consciousness, so black is associated with ignorance, lack of awareness, or the unconscious.

Black indicates negation and absence of pranic energy. It shades lighter, brighter colors into lower vibrations and robs them of energy. Black is often seen in the aura of individuals with serious illness or astral possession. Black that glows with crimson red is a vicious combination. Deep bluish-black obscuring the face indicates imminent death.

- **Positive black qualities:** rest, relaxation, sleep, stillness, withdrawal.

- **Negative black qualities:** hatred, hopeless grief, oppression, gloom, pessimism, depression, malice, revenge, evil, malevolence, illness, astral possession.

Brown—Earth

Brown is an elemental, down-to-earth color, the hue of soil and tree bark. Brown in the aura indicates business acumen, industry, organization, orderly management, and desire for gain and accumulation. It is associated with growth, effort, and desire to accomplish and succeed. Any mundane, secular affairs are enhanced with brown in the energy field.

- **Clear brown:** industrious accumulation, strength, reliability, consistency, painstaking perseverance, earthiness.

- **Muddy brown:** negativity, stubbornness, inflexibility, rigidity, miserliness, greed, avarice, corruption.

Gray—Depression

Gray auras are persistent people who work hard to get tasks done. They are often lone wolves who want to live life on their own terms. Gray in the aura often indicates illness, grief, sorrow, and loss. Blackish-gray is a dull, heavy vibration. Leaden gray indicates fear, cowardice, doubt of previously held beliefs, and indecisiveness. Murky gray indicates negativity, depression, hopelessness, negativity, deceit, or decay of mind, body, and/or organs. Silver brings greater sparkle.

Anomalies in the Auric Field

You may see many unusual flecks, steaks, bars, or clouds in an energy field. Here are a few examples:

- Lightning streaks of red or bright yellow—mental agitation or conflict.

- Gray bars flashing around throat or joints—taking prescription drugs.

- Black and red flecks bouncing around heart and lungs—addiction to hard drugs such as cocaine or heroin.

- Khaki and murky green with red and orange flecks—infected area of body.

- Whirling, dark, muddy purple flecks throughout aura—homosexuality.

- Flecks of muddy orange in abdominal area—food allergies.

- Streaks and spires flashing muddy yellow around head and spinal column—fear (a "yellow streak").

- A shrunken aura, with gray blobs around eyes, nose, throat and top of head, along with a red blob in heart center that shrinks in and out—alcoholism.

- Brown or gray blobs next to head—astral possession or oppression (see page 144 for more information).

- White balls of light next to head—spiritual guides, angels, or departed loved ones.

- Gray or brown spots—illness in that area of the body.

- Dark hole on top of head—migraine headaches, or communication from the other side.

♦   Little hooks of light scattered throughout the field—a leader, director, or overseer of large groups of people.

♦   Bright green coming in on left side—starting over or rejuvenation.

♦   Gold coming in on left side—remodeling a home or new creativity.

In the next chapter, you will learn how to heal lower vibrational entities and other external influences that may deplete or damage your energy field.

Part III

❧

Cleansing Your Energy Field

9

Healing Environ-Mental Static

ಬಬ

Healing Your Auric Atmosphere

"Light, even though it passes through pollution, is not polluted."

—Augustine[1]

Boxing champion Mike Tyson and television actress Robin Givens were married on February 7, 1988, after Robin found she was pregnant. That was a year of infidelity, spousal abuse, restraining orders, and car crashes. Tyson bragged that he threw his greatest punch at the woman he had vowed to love forever: "She flew backward, hitting every [bleeping] wall in the apartment."

In an interview with Barbara Walters on September 30, 1988, Givens described life with Tyson as "torture...pure hell...worse than anything I could possibly imagine."[2] Meanwhile, Tyson sat right next to her, silently stroking her neck. Two days later, Tyson allegedly became violent. Givens filed for divorce. The fighter labeled her a "gold-digger" and "slime of the slime." They divorced on Valentine's Day, 1989.

On November 5, 2004, on the Oprah Winfrey Show, Robin reported that during her marriage Mike beat her and threatened to kill her. She feared Mike might murder her, yet she stayed with him anyway.

Oprah Winfrey reminisced about a time she accepted an invitation to visit Mike and Robin's fabulous mansion. When Oprah arrived, she sensed something was really off. Robin asked her to stay overnight, but the atmosphere was so tense that Oprah refused the invitation. But when Oprah arrived at the train station, she had missed her train. She returned to the Tyson home to spend the night. However, the energy there was so terrible that Oprah left in the middle of the night and did not return.[3]

Have you ever sensed such dreadful feelings when you entered someone's home? Have you ever been drained by negative energies? Do you think of certain people as "black holes"—no matter how far you bend over backward to please them, it is never enough? Do overly needy, clingy people seek your attention? Have you ever felt claustrophobic at crowded events—as though the jam-packed sea of humanity were closing in on you?

Many detrimental influences can encroach upon your auric field. You may be seriously depleted, weakened, afflicted, or even wounded by intensely negative vibrations from:

1. People around you.
2. Your loved ones.
3. Your coworkers.
4. Your peers.
5. The vibratory atmosphere at home or work.
6. The atmosphere in crowded areas such as subways, trains, planes, theaters, restaurants, bars, schools, stadiums, or concert halls.
7. The atmosphere of hospitals, mental institutions, or prisons.
8. Lower vibrational energies from the astral plane.

What is the nature of these subtle energies, and how do they affect you adversely?

The Astral-Mental World

Please refer to Figure 9a on the following page, which shows various aspects of the astral/mental plane. The two basic parts of this realm are your individual subconscious mind, which you read about on page 59, and the collective subconscious mind of humanity.

The Astral/Mental World

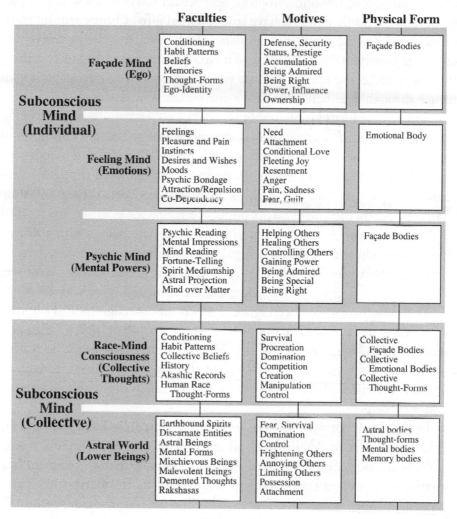

		Faculties	Motives	Physical Form
Subconscious Mind (Individual)	**Façade Mind (Ego)**	Conditioning Habit Patterns Beliefs Memories Thought-Forms Ego-Identity	Defense, Security Status, Prestige Accumulation Being Admired Being Right Power, Influence Ownership	Façade Bodies
	Feeling Mind (Emotions)	Feelings Pleasure and Pain Instincts Desires and Wishes Moods Psychic Bondage Attraction/Repulsion Co-Dependency	Need Attachment Conditional Love Fleeting Joy Resentment Anger Pain, Sadness Fear, Guilt	Emotional Body
	Psychic Mind (Mental Powers)	Psychic Reading Mental Impressions Mind Reading Fortune-Telling Spirit Mediumship Astral Projection Mind over Matter	Helping Others Healing Others Controlling Others Gaining Power Being Admired Being Special Being Right	Façade Bodies

Subconscious Mind (Collective)	**Race-Mind Consciousness (Collective Thoughts)**	Conditioning
		Habit Patterns
		Collective Beliefs
		History
		Akashic Records
		Human Race
		  Thought-Forms
			Survival
			Procreation
			Domination
			Competition
			Creation
			Manipulation
			Control
				Collective
				  Façade Bodies
				Collective
				  Emotional Bodies
				Collective
				  Thought-Forms

	Astral World (Lower Beings)	Earthbound Spirits Discarnate Entities Astral Beings Mental Forms Mischievous Beings Malevolent Beings Demented Thoughts Rakshasas	Fear, Survival Domination Control Frightening Others Annoying Others Limiting Others Possession Attachment	Astral bodies Thought-forms Mental bodies Memory bodies

Figure 9a.

Your *façade mind* consists of false, limited ego-constructs by which you identify yourself. Built of encrusted habits so deeply ingrained that they crystallize into solid form, the façade body is often perceived as armor, a protective covering of defensiveness. It is entirely illusory and can be healed through prayer and love.

The *psychic mind* consists of faculties of subtle mental perceptions—talents not necessarily understood or accepted. However, these talents can be developed. Some psychics have true spiritual gifts. Others acquire mental powers from the astral/mental plane. Predictions may be extremely accurate or grossly inaccurate, because mental/emotional states, in continual flux, have no lasting reality. Because you are the one who creates your own future through free will, changing your beliefs will change your destiny. Therefore, your future is malleable.

The *race-mind consciousness* is comprised of collective thoughts of humanity—an accumulation of societal beliefs, habits, and conditions born of communal, social, religious, political, and national thought-forms (beliefs so intense that they solidify into form). Often these beliefs are shared by nearly the entire earth's population.

The *entity world* consists of invisible disincarnate beings with a slower, denser vibration than spiritual beings. Astral entities are often perceived by those sensitive to feeling subtle vibrations, and it is essential for sensitives to learn how to deal with these energies.

The entity world has been ignored by countless religions and philosophies that deny its existence out of fear. Many people do not want to give credence to the negative side of life. However, the entity world is neither frightening nor negative. It simply needs healing. It is vital to learn how to heal experiences of the entity world, because such experiences exist and cannot be denied.

In this book you will learn to become so self-empowered that you are no longer subject to detrimental influences from the astral/mental world. By using the power of the spoken word through affirmation, you can heal negative energies and take command over your life. In the next few chapters you will learn powerful affirmative healing prayers that can profoundly transform your energy field within just a few minutes.

Astral Auric Intrusion

When Gladys McCoy, master dowser from Fayetteville, Arkansas, and cofounder of the Ozark Research Institute,[4] traveled from Vermont to Arkansas one summer, she stayed in a crowded motel. The only space available was a room for people with disabilities that was partially underground. When Gladys entered the room, she felt a murky, dense atmospheric energy.

As soon as her husband, Harold, left the room to get a soda, an earth-bound spirit suddenly jumped onto Gladys and attached itself to her energy field. Although she felt threatened and afraid, Gladys spun slowly in a circle and chanted repeatedly aloud, "I AM a child of God, and therefore the demonic forces cannot harm me." When her husband returned, she was still visibly shaken. Harold, a master healer, helped Gladys settle down. He soothed her auric field and brought her energies back into alignment. The room then felt fine for the rest of the night, and they drove home safely.

A healthy, active, strong, wiry man in his 80s, Mr. D trimmed the trees and shrubbery around Gladys and Harold McCoy's healing center[5] in Fayetteville. Mr. D had led a fascinating life as an activist. Whenever there was a cause, he joined in. One day he moved into a tiny retirement apartment to write his memoirs.

Just two weeks later, Gladys was shocked to discover that Mr. D had suddenly become severely incapacitated. His body, in enormous pain, was contorted, twisted, and bent over with a seemingly major arthritic condition. Finally, he seemed to lose all hope, as though his spirit had left him.

At the end of his rope, Mr. D hobbled to Gladys's center on crutches, where he received a healing on her massage table. She asked him to draw a diagram of his apartment, and she used her pendulum to locate detrimental energies in his building. As she was clearing the adverse energies, suddenly she saw a vision of a Native American Indian with disabilities. He was bent and gnarled, dragging himself around with two forked sticks bound with rawhide to his upper arms, which he used as crutches.

Gladys discovered that the Indian was fond of Mr. D and had taken possession of his body. She spoke lovingly to the Indian and explained that he was hurting Mr. D. She asked the Indian to leave the premises. The Indian was unwilling to leave the earth plane, but he was willing to leave the apartment. So he moved on.

Within one week, Mr. D was totally well, back to his normal, active lifestyle, climbing trees with his chainsaw. It turned out that his apartment was located along the Trail of Tears in an area with many Indian mounds. If you are sensitive, you can feel the sadness and sorrow in the atmosphere in that region.

How did Mr. D become possessed by the Indian? And why would any soul possess a living human?

Earthbound Spirits

Undoubtedly you are aware of the "near-death experience" (NDE) reported by thousands of people who have temporarily flatlined (meaning that they stopped breathing and their EEG or brain-wave activity ceased). Survivors of NDEs often report leaving their body during the flatline period and moving toward a divine light of immeasurable beauty and glory. I am firmly convinced that NDEs are real and that they reveal what happens after death.

At death, souls leave their physical bodies and move into the divine light. Then they have a "life review," in which their life is played back like a movie. They see this movie not only from their own perspective, but also from the viewpoint of every other person they ever encountered. In other words, the soul walks in the shoes of every person that soul ever met in that lifetime, and the soul sees how it affected each person.

However, some souls do not enter this divine light after death. These souls have dense, nearly impenetrable auras and get trapped in an astral prison of their own making. They cannot see the spiritual light and divine landscape around them. Blind to the brilliant colors and hues of the celestial realm, deaf to the music of the spheres, and alone in the midst of loved ones whom they refuse to see, they dwell in a land of self-made hell.

Why would any soul choose blindness instead of the beautiful divine light after death?

1. Perhaps the person had an unexpected, accidental, or violent death. When this happens, the soul suddenly catapults out of the body and does not even realize it is dead.

2. The soul might be lost, confused, and wandering in a dazed state. This can happen in cases of Alzheimer's disease, senility, or heavy drug use just before death.

3. Perhaps the individual does not believe in God, in a light, or in an afterlife. Convinced that nothing exists after death, the soul is prevented from seeing or entering the light.

4. If the person is arrogant or stubborn, then the soul might not accept help from departed loved ones in the tunnel who are ushering it into the divine light.

Why a Departed Spirit Becomes Earthbound

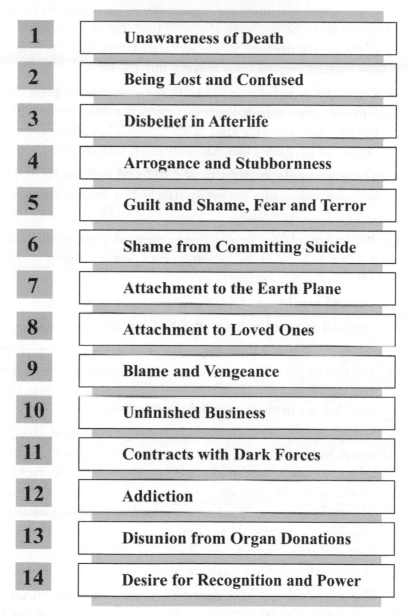

1	**Unawareness of Death**
2	**Being Lost and Confused**
3	**Disbelief in Afterlife**
4	**Arrogance and Stubbornness**
5	**Guilt and Shame, Fear and Terror**
6	**Shame from Committing Suicide**
7	**Attachment to the Earth Plane**
8	**Attachment to Loved Ones**
9	**Blame and Vengeance**
10	**Unfinished Business**
11	**Contracts with Dark Forces**
12	**Addiction**
13	**Disunion from Organ Donations**
14	**Desire for Recognition and Power**

Figure 9b.

5. The individual was constantly told how sinful he/she is and that he/she was born in sin. Such a soul may feel unworthy to go into the divine light. The person may also believe that at death he/she will enter the "Pearly Gates" and meet St. Peter. Then, once the big book of sins is read, the soul imagines it might be condemned to hellfire and damnation. Such fear can prevent the soul from moving into the light.

6. The soul may feel shame and guilt due to committing suicide. However, even suicide souls can enter the light after death. But they have a unique kind of life review. They see what their life would have been like, had they continued to live.

7. The soul may be overly attached to loved ones on earth, or have loved ones who are overly attached to the departed soul and are holding it back.

8. The soul may be overly attached to the earth plane or to material things. It may continue to haunt a home or other building—sometimes for centuries.

9. The soul may be angry, blaming, and seeking vengeance.

10. The soul may feel it has unfinished business to accomplish before it is ready to move on.

11. The soul might believe it made a contract, pact, or agreement with dark forces and therefore thinks it cannot move into the light. Yet, it can choose the light at any time.

12. Perhaps the person suffered an addiction to alcohol, drugs, sex, or food. Without a body, the soul cannot continue that habit after death, so it might attempt to attach to a living human to continue to enjoy pleasures of the flesh. As a result, a living human may become oppressed or possessed by that soul. Who is susceptible to astral possession? People suffering from addiction, depression, illness, an accident, alcoholism, or those who are under anesthesia or other weakened states.

13. The individual may have signed an organ donor card without considering the consequences. An overly attached deceased soul, clinging to the physical body, may feel terrorized when

the body is dismembered. However, if the person perceives him-/herself as a spiritual being temporarily inhabiting this physical shell, then donating organs will not prevent the soul from moving on.

14. During his/her life, the person may have been frustrated by his/her attempts at earthly fame, recognition, and power. Therefore in the afterlife the soul may attach itself to a living human medium or channeler. This spirit may give the medium a fake, impressive name, such as a Biblical name, and then achieve celebrity through speaking or writing messages through that medium. This is a "faker spirit."

I believe the afterlife consists of your own heaven or hell conceived by your own thought-forms. Thus gifted clairvoyants cannot perceive any plane of existence that can be described as "hell," other than the dark defensive energy fields of those souls who generate muddy auras.

Earthbound spirits, discarnate entities, astral entities, ghosts, poltergeists (mischievous ghosts that rattle windows and doors and turn televisions and lights on and off), phantoms, specters—these are all names for spirits living in the astral world.

One definition given for the term *exorcism* is "the driving out of evil spirits." However, most entities are not "evil," although they lower the vibrational energy of the atmosphere. They are usually lost, confused, and ignorant. Only a small percentage have malicious, malevolent, or mischievous intentions. "Driving out spirits" is not a permanent solution. If you force a spirit to leave, it will return later, or it will haunt or possess someone else, such as a neighbor, a child, a pet, or your mother-in-law.

All entities have one thing in common: they need healing. If they are willing to move into the light, or if you can convince them to move into the light, then they will never influence you or your loved ones again.

Albert Marsh from Los Angeles reports his experiences with healing entities:

It's quick and easy and works. For many, just saying "healed and forgiven" a few times does it. When I first got into this teaching, I had a lot of entity action, and used the prayer several times a day when I felt down or ungrounded. Over time, I guess the entities just caught

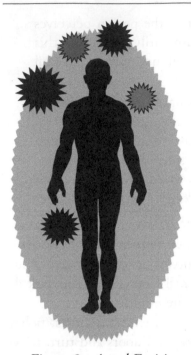

Figure 9c. Astral Entities

on that they were wasting their time with me, and laid off. Now I'm almost always clear. When I feel entity influence, the change is so obvious that I heal it immediately with the prayer.

The prayers that follow will help you send these entities into the divine light. These are spoken lovingly and are directed toward the entity needing healing. Once you use these astral-entity healing prayers, the energy field of your surroundings immediately lifts. It becomes lighter and less dense.

Important Note: All the prayers and affirmations in this book are to be spoken audibly in a powerful, clear voice. These can be used to heal yourself or to heal others. Speak aloud with conviction, confidence, and certainty. (You can order a CD of *35 Spiritual Healing Prayers* at *www.divinerevelation.org*. You can also learn and use a total of 243 healing prayers in my book *Instant Healing*.)

Astral Entity Healing Prayers

Prayer to Heal and Forgive Entities
(healing prayer to send entities into the light)

Beloved ones, you are unified with the truth of your being.
You are lifted in divine love.
You are forgiven of all guilt and shame.
You are healed and released
From loss, pain, confusion, and fear.
Divine love and light fill and surround you now.
Attachment to the earth no longer binds you.
You are free to go into the divine light now.
Go now in peace and love.

One of my students asked my online prayer group to pray for his deceased mother, Ovella. Soon afterward, I received the following email: *"I want to thank all of you who prayed for my mother. During my meditation this morning, I received a message from her that she had at last moved on. She related to me that she has been concerned for all of her children, especially my younger sister. I assured her that we are fine and will be okay, and she acknowledged that as true. She also reports that it is so beautiful where she is now and she feels such joy and peace. She sounded happy and peaceful. She has finally moved on to her deserved period of rest."*

Chant to Heal and Lift Entities

(healing chant for healing entities and lifting the vibratory atmosphere)

I call upon Holy Spirit
To lovingly heal any and all dear ones
That are wise to heal at this time.
Dear ones, you are lovingly bless-ed, forgiven, and released,
Into the love, light, and wholeness of the universal God Consciousness.
Bless-ed, forgiven, and released,
Into the love, light, and wholeness of the universal God Consciousness.

(Repeat the last two lines until you feel the entities have gone into the light.)

Albert Marsh from Los Angeles reports:

One time I healed a poltergeist, and it was absolutely no big deal. A family moved into a house and, soon after, weird things started to happen, and the family was very fearful. I said the healing prayer for the entity and then forgot about it. Several weeks later I asked about the haunting. I found out the weirdness had stopped suddenly and the family was happy and at peace again. As simply as that. No priests or holy water or Bibles—no drama. In fact they had gone the priest route and it had no effect whatsoever on the problem.

E.T. Astral Healing Prayer

(for healing malevolent extraterrestrial entities and outer-space
beings and for clearing alien abductees)

Dear ones, you are all healed and forgiven.
You are merged, unified, filled, and surrounded
With your own universal cosmic divine nature.
You are merged, unified, filled, and surrounded
With universal cosmic divine love.
You are merged, unified, filled, and surrounded
With universal cosmic divine light.
Dear ones, you are lovingly bless-ed, forgiven, and released,
Into the love, light, and wholeness
Of the universal God Consciousness.
You are all free from fear, pain, and from the earth's
And all other planetary vibrations,
In this and all other dimensions.
I call upon Jesus and Sananda,
The universal cosmic Christ Consciousness,
To take you all to your own right places of expression.
Go in peace and in love.
I now cut any and all psychic ties between
(insert name of person here) *and any dear ones.*
These psychic ties are now lovingly cut, lifted, loved
Healed, released, dissolved, and completely let go.
Thank you God, and SO IT IS.

Mass Astral Healing

Sometimes you may sense that more than one entity needs healing. Then ask your higher self, "Is there a mass here for healing?" If you receive a Yes response, then you know a group of earthbound spirits needs healing. Anytime there is a great tragedy and many souls are lost, such as a terrorist attack, earthquake, or tsunami, mass healings are required.

You can then say, "I welcome you all in love and light. You are all healed and forgiven." Then just continue to say, "Healed and forgiven" repeatedly until you sense the healing is done. Ask if the healing is complete; if you get a No, repeat the phrase again until you get a Yes.

This same simple affirmation is very effective for clearing a building of astral entities or hauntings. Open all the cupboards and closets in the building and then walk through every room. In every nook and cranny hold your hands out to bless the space as you chant, "Healed and forgiven" repeatedly, until the entire house is cleared.

You may also use the following prayer for healing massive groups of entities from natural disasters, war zones, and so forth:

> *I call upon the Holy Spirit to cut any and all psychic ties*
> *Between myself and any and all dear ones*
> *That have come for healing at this time.*
> *I now visualize a beauteous golden dome*
> *Of protective divine love and light high above this place.*
> *The Beautiful Many divine beings of light and "I AMs"*
> *Now welcome any and all entities in need of healing now.*
> *These entities are now healed and lifted into the light now.*
> *Beloved ones, you are all unified with the truth of your being.*
> *You are lifted in divine love.*
> *You are forgiven of all guilt and shame.*
> *You are healed and released*
> *From loss, pain, confusion, and fear.*
> *Divine love and light fills and surrounds you now.*
> *Attachment to the earth no longer binds you.*
> *You are free to go into the divine light now.*
> *Go now in peace and love.*
> *I now give thanks that part of our assignment on earth*
> *Is to help dissipate the astral cloud to clear the way*
> *For the earth's vibrational lifting and enlightenment.*
> *Thank you God, and SO IT IS.*

Healing Psychic Vampires

The lore of vampirism has a corresponding reality in everyday life. Do you have friends or relatives who act like vampires? These are needy people who drain your energy and suck it dry. They demand your attention, love, time, and life-force. In fact, they are bottomless pits into which you keep tossing your energy. Enabling these people by always saying yes to them will not heal them.

Energy vampires can absorb pranic power through hugging, patting, or grabbing. Some speak softly and timidly, forcing you to extend your

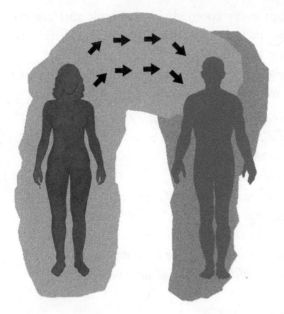

Figure 9d. Energy Vampirism

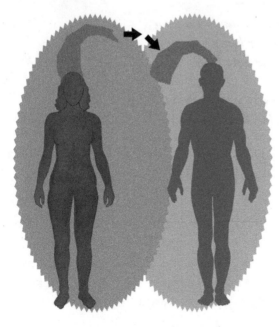

Figure 9e. Psychic Hooks

energy field into theirs. Others get in your face, speak too loudly, or stand too close, right inside your aura. Some open their eyes wide to draw in energy. Others phone or arrive at odd hours, rattling on endlessly, whining about their woes. Or they shoot energy daggers from their eyes.

People are not the only energy vampires. Lower beings from the astral world that see and feel your light, love, and power may attempt to install psychic hooks in your auric field. Energy suckers are always on the lookout for "spigots" to hook into. Once the pump opens, spiritual energy drains from your auric field. That is why it is essential to maintain spiritual protection. (See Chapter 10.)

If you are plagued by psychic vampirism, remember that your deep soul has asked for this experience so you may learn and understand this experience and help others lift themselves out of such deplorable situations.

The following prayers can heal psychic vampirism and hooks.

Psychic Vampire Healing Prayer

I AM held in the arms of God. I AM cradled in God's love.
I AM held in the palm of God's hand.
God brings me peace, light, wholeness, and blessings.
I AM filled with divine light and love.
I AM filled with radiance, purity, and wholeness.
I AM wholeness and oneness.
Where there is wholeness, there are no parts.
Where there is oneness, there is no psychic vampire,
Psychic drain, psychic sponge, or psychic energy loss.
When there is oneness, there is no loss or gain.
I trust in this oneness and know that I AM that oneness.
I AM the true beauteous nature of God beingness.
Thank you God, and SO IT IS.

Psychic Hook Healing

My heart now melts in divine love.
I AM a beloved child of God.
I AM filled with the light of God.
There is no energy that I need fear.
For the Lord my God is with me wherever I go.
There is no energy that has any control over me.
For the Lord my God is with me wherever I go.
There is no entity that can place hooks in me.
For I AM a God-being living in human form, in human flesh.
I AM a being of great light, of great good,
Of great glory, and of great purity.
And God's love fills and surrounds me now.
Thank you God, and SO IT IS.

Healing Ancestral Influences

Your blood relatives, living and dead, can cause your aura to shrink or be bound by ancestral ties, ropes, karmic bonds, and other binding attachments. Abusive words and deeds from family members have lasting devastating effects on your energy field.

Well-meaning relatives might smother you with what they define as "love," which is, in reality, codependency, psychic vampirism, or psychic attack. They may believe that warning you of this perilous world and your likelihood of failure will prevent you from harm. They might offer sage advice about how ridiculous you are for trying to achieve your impossible dreams and goals. Or they might remind you how people are laughing at you for following your heart and doing something that does not fit the "norm."

If you feel your relatives tugging on or binding up your energy field, holding you back from achieving your dreams, then use these prayers.

Familial Healing Prayer

I know now and I affirm that my relatives are lifted up
In the cleansing, healing light of God's vibration,
They now live in this beauteous divine sphere of light,
Protected, whole and secure in the light of God.
I know now that all my relations
Are safe, secure, and at peace.
My relatives have no effect whatsoever
Upon my God Consciousness now.
All psychic ties, connections, karmic bonds, and binding ties
Between myself and my relations are now lovingly
Dissolved, cut, released, blessed, healed, let go,
And lifted into the light of God now, and they are gone.
I AM now free of these karmic bonds and binding ties,
I AM no longer subject to psychic attacks,
Psychic vampirism, or psychic influence.
I AM now free of all seeming attacks,
And they are but pappus fluff.
They have no effect whatsoever.
I AM free. I AM filled with God's holy presence.
I AM a radiant being of light,
Filled with God's holy vibration.
My energy field vibrates and radiates the light of God.
All is perfect and all is well.
Thank you God, and SO IT IS.

Deceased Ancestor Healing

(for healing binding affects from old ancestral binding ties)

There is no energy from this world or any other world
That can lessen or diminish my God Consciousness.
All energies from this world and from any other world
That do not reflect the truth of my being
Are now lovingly lifted, healed, blessed, released, let go,
And filled with the light of God.
All seeming influence from past times,
Any ancestors that are not of God,
And any and all other dear ones that are not of God—
All these beings are now lovingly and permanently
Lifted into the light of God's love and truth.
Beloved ones, you are united with the truth of your being.
You are lifted in divine love.
God's radiant love, radiant light and radiant power
Fill and surround you now
With immeasurable peace and immeasurable love.
You are now free from this earthly vibration.
You are free to go into God's holy presence and divine light now.
Go in peace, dear ones, and go in love.
Thank you God, and SO IT IS.

Healing Reptilians

Beings called *reptilians* are working with dark energies from the astral world. These beings incarnate on earth with malevolent intentions to cause confusion, drain energy, and confound light beings and light workers who are lifting the planet. This so-called *reptilian energy* is a dark, astral energy—not E.T. energy. It is an extra-dimensional energy of lower aspects of the astral world, where demonic beings reside.

Some reptilians have been humans in the past. Others have never been human. These reptilian energies have enticing and enchanting powers. Certain gurus with reptilian energy build a special mystique and glamour around themselves. Others have a psychic draining or psychic vampire energy.

Use the following prayer if you suspect you are dealing with a reptilian:

Reptilian Healing Prayer

I now let go of all fear. I know that in any situation,
No matter what, I now use my power of discernment
To heal and release any seeming reptilian influence now.
I now transform my energy field through the power of God's love.
All psychic bonds between myself and seeming reptilian energies
Are now lovingly lifted, healed, untied, cut, loved, dissolved, released,
And completely let go into the light of God now.
There is no longer any influence from reptilian energies now.
Dear seeming reptilian ones,
You are unified with the truth of your being.
You are lifted in divine love.
You are filled with the light of God.
You are filled with divine truth.
You are filled with forgiveness.
You are free from all contracts and obligations
That you have made with seeming dark forces or energies.
You are free to experience your true nature of being,
And to let go of all fear, glamour, illusion,
Enchantment, mystique, and ego-enticements.
You are free to be who you truly are.
Open your heart to God's love, God's light, and God's truth.
Let go, let God, and be at peace, dear ones.
Thank you God, and SO IT IS.

In the next chapter, you will practice powerful methods for spiritual self-defense and preventing energy drain from external influences.

10

Are You a Psychic Sponge?

ၿၿ

Developing Auric Protection and Self-Authority

"They who have light in themselves will not revolve as satellites."
—Seneca[1]

Amy Levinson, a Tarot reader from New York, says, *"I get so drained from dealing with all these people. I feel like a wet mop being dragged through the mud all day. Like energy vampires are sucking me dry all day long. By the end of the day, all I can do is collapse onto my bed. I get so exhausted."*

Unfortunately, many people sensitive to subtle energies are blind to fundamental necessities—breathing, diet, exercise, and prana. Some psychics or healers tend to categorically ignore the health of their own auric field. Others simply have no clue about closing off their aura or opening to the flow of divine energy during their work. We all need to practice "aural hygiene." Just as we have a daily routine for cleansing our body, it is essential to add a few practices each day to keep our aura free from impurities and anomalies.

A weak, collapsed, or punctured aura is particularly susceptible to lower energies, astral possession, psychic vampirism, difficult experiences, mental illness, and even disease. We travel in our energy field as a turtle travels in

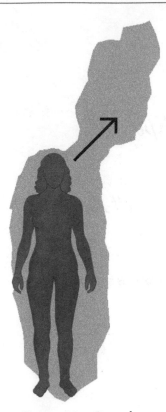

Figure 10a. Detachment

its shell. When our shell is cracked or broken, we flounder about unprotected, unsafe, and insecure in unwholesome environments. You may not see yourself with a cracked auric shield, but if you can relate to the following complaint, then you might be what I call a *psychic sponge.*

Stuart Mark Van Niekerk from Scotland writes, "*When I get involved with work, people, or relationships, I am like a psychic sponge that soaks up everything in the ether. I notice that my aura weakens. I might feel strange energies and struggle with anger or fear. I can sense the feeling coming on, but am unsure what is the best way to dwell in the light, no matter what situation. Any suggestions?*"

Psychic sponges absorb vibrational energies from their surroundings, just as a sponge absorbs water. Their auras—open, oversensitive, and vulnerable—are subject to all energies, even harmful ones. Here is my prescription for all psychic sponges: Study this chapter and use the affirmations daily. In this way, you will build an impermeable aura of great strength and fortitude. With regular practice, you can become a fountainhead of unlimited energy rather than a psychic sponge. Once your powerful pranic energy is overflowing, share it with others.

Janet Rittington of Louisville, Kentucky, states, "*I felt impeded by energetic influences and drains. I was confused/depleted/clouded/tired, and it was not bodily tiredness, poor food, or other simple explanations. Using Dr. Susan's methods, I learned how to clear these energies and the proof was in the results. Now I clear myself regularly with these healing prayers.*"

What aggravates psychic sponge syndrome? Psychic sponges are often well-meaning, sensitive people who simply do not know how to keep their auras closed. Some of them may suffer weakness, gullibility, self-deprecation, instability, or susceptibility. Impressionable and naive, they might run after glamorous gurus. They may lack discernment or misjudge character. Perhaps they construe astral experiences as true spiritual experiences. Maybe they meditate too long or too often. They might be ungrounded, even detached from their bodies (Figure 10a). They may engage in astral travel or other occult practices without safeguards. Perhaps they are obsessed with things detrimental to their spiritual evolution, or consumed by opinions of others.

The quality of the love vibration that you radiate will determine how strong your energy field is. A powerful auric field is safe from peril, immune from disease, unaffected by talebearers, and impervious to naysayers.

Auric Self-Defense

It is said that an ounce of prevention is worth a pound of cure. There is no truer statement to describe strengthening the human energy field. Practicing daily "aural hygiene" is essential to our well-being. By simply speaking affirmations of inner divine protection just a few times daily, I guarantee your aura will become stronger and more powerful; eventually it can even become invincible.

I use affirmations of spiritual protection every day and have done so since 1986. I recommend saying such affirmations audibly whenever you leave your home, before you go to sleep, before you meditate, before going to a meeting, when you enter a crowd, before entering a low vibrational atmosphere, before and after meeting a client, before meeting with your boss or your mother-in-law, and in any intimidating situation.

In these affirmations you will close your aura to the lower vibrational levels of mind and the astral world, and you will open your aura to God and the spiritual plane.

Important Note: All the prayers and affirmations in this book are to be spoken in a powerful, clear voice. When you use the words "I AM," say the phrase as though your higher self is saying it. These affirmative prayers can be used to heal yourself or to heal others. Speak audibly with conviction, confidence, and certainty.

Self-Authority Affirmation
(for greater self-reliance, confidence, and inner strength)
I AM in control. I AM one with God.
I AM the only authority in my life.

I AM divinely protected by the light of my being.
I close off my aura and body of light
To the lower astral levels of mind
And I open to the spiritual world,
Now and forevermore.
Thank you God, and SO IT IS.

Stephen Hesch from Madison, Wisconsin, sent me this email: *"I recite the Prayer of Self-Authority from Susan's book daily, and have for many months now, and it has had a profound, positive effect on how I think and view the Universe. I speak this prayer from the 'I AM' self, not the ego-based, personality-based self. I highly recommend this prayer to anyone seeking a better understanding of his or her true nature."*

God-Authority Affirmation

(an alternative to the Self-Authority Affirmation)
The God in me is in control.
The God in me is the only authority in my life.
I close off my aura and body of light
To all but my own God-self and consciousness
Now and forevermore.
Thank you God, and SO IT IS.

Prayer of Protection

(for divine protection and divine love; used in Unity Church of Christianity)
The light of God surrounds me.
The love of God enfolds me.
The power of God protects me.
The presence of God watches over me.
Wherever I AM, God is, and all is well.

Pillar of Light Visualization

One powerful way to create a protective aura of divine light is to visualize one. Many people imagine a sphere, bubble, or column of light permeating, surrounding, and protecting them. Please refer to Figure 10b and then practice the visualization exercise that follows.

Close your eyes and imagine a beauteous sphere of protective divine light above your head, of whatever color you wish. Then see a ray of that light streaming down through the midline of your body, all the way from the top of your head to the tips of your toes. Visualize this light ray vibrating and radiating from your energy centers, filling your entire energy field with a column of divine light.

This beauteous light fills your energy field with divine love, power, energy, invincibility, joy, happiness, and fulfillment. Feel this divine light vibrating and radiating within you and around you. You are divinely protected by the light of your being.

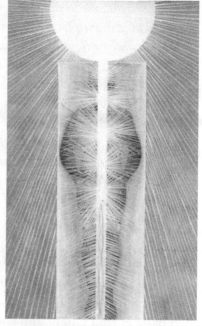

Figure 10b. Pillar of Light

Staying Grounded

There are many powerful ways to stay grounded, centered, balanced, and in control. Walking around barefoot or imagining a cord reaching deep into the earth—this is not being grounded in Spirit. Grounding is uniting with God, with the true nature of your being. Here is an affirmation to help you stay grounded and centered in Spirit:

Grounded in Spirit

I AM blessed and beloved. My heart soars into Spirit.
I AM a beloved being of great power,
Great light, energy, and glory.
I AM a beauteous being, a radiant being of light.
I AM lifted into the light of God.
I AM established and grounded
In the true nature of my being. God is within me.
God lives, breathes, moves, and has its being in me and through me.
I AM a beloved being of great power,

Great light, and great glory.
I AM filled with love, filled with peace, and filled with power.
God's healing light fills and surrounds me now.
God's healing energy lifts my vibration now
And fills me with peace.
I AM a beloved being of great light and great energy.
I trust in this and know that I AM loved.
I AM filled with love and light.
God's radiant sphere of divine energy
Now grounds me in God's holy presence.
This is the holy presence that I AM grounded in.
Thank you God, and SO IT IS.

Auric Cleansing and Healing

Healing and cleansing your energy field can fill your life with peace, joy, prosperity, and light. Your aura can be cleansed and augmented with two basic energies: light and sound. The following affirmations transform your energy field with light, and speaking these affirmations aloud positively affects your energy field through sound. To learn more about the ascended masters mentioned in these prayers, such as Babaji and Saint Germain, read my book *Ascension*.

Let There Be Light Prayer

Let there be light. The loving, empowering,
White, golden, violet, pink, green, and blue
Healing, soothing, energizing, divine light
Of Jesus, Babaji, the Holy Spirit, and
(insert name of your deity here)
In and through this God-filled, healing, empowerment
Aura cleansing and healing session and situation now,
For the highest good of myself, and all others concerned.
(Repeat all above verses at least three times.)
Thank you God, and SO IT IS.

White Fire Affirmation

I AM now lovingly lifted, healed and cleansed.
In the white fire of the Holy Spirit

And God Consciousness,
And the violet cleansing flame of Saint Germain,
Under God's grace, in God's own wise and perfect ways.
Thank you God, and SO IT IS.

Golden Healing Prayer

I AM now lovingly filled, lifted, and surrounded
With the golden healing substance of God Consciousness.
I AM now filled with God's love,
God's light, and God's truth.
God now fills my aura and body of light
With this golden healing substance,
Which closes the doors of both
My physical and subtle bodies
To the lower astral levels of mind
And instead attunes me to God Consciousness.
This golden healing substance now heals and lifts me.
It awakens my awareness to God Consciousness
Within me and within all of creation, now.
I AM healed, and I AM more fully attuned
To God within me, and in all creation.
I lovingly awaken to greater awareness
Of God within me right now.
Thank you God, and SO IT IS.

Auric First-Aid

Your aura can be compromised in many ways. Psychic vampires can suck energy from your auric field. Drugs, alcohol, cigarettes, or other addictive substances can damage your aura. Improper food, shallow breathing, negative thinking, or stress can diminish your energy field. Playing with the occult without safeguards and protections can invite lower energies that pierce holes in your field. Here are some powerful affirmations for repairing damaged, injured energy fields.

Three of the affirmations in this chapter ("Closing Holes," "Calling Back Parts Into Wholeness of Self," and "Releasing Agreements") are part of a group of healing prayers called Divine Mother's Vibrational Tools, created by Connie Huebner.[2]

Closing Holes[3]

I call upon Jesus Christ,
Lord Sananda and Divine Mother
To close all doors, openings, holes, portals, and gateways
Anywhere in my multidimensional energy system,
To all limited planes, planets,
Domains, dimensions, spheres, realms
And places anywhere in creation.
(You can elaborate here and close holes to any or all situations,
people, events, and so forth that are "holding" you.)
These holes, doors, openings, portals, and gateways
Are now closed and sealed
In the name and through the power of Jesus Christ,
In the name and through the power of Lord Sananda,
In the name and through the power of Divine Mother.
Any energetic configurations or attracting mechanisms
Around these now closed holes and openings
Are now dismantled, dissolved and released.
And I AM opening fully in Wholeness of Divine Love,
Aligning with Wholeness of Divine Truth,
Allowing Wholeness of Divine Grace.
I AM aligned with Truth...
Thank you God and SO IT IS.

Calling Back Parts Into Wholeness of Self[4]

(Make the following statements with strong intention and knowing
that they are so.) *I call back to my Self all parts of my self that have ever been*
separated, isolated, fragmented, lost, or given away. (You can elaborate here
and call back parts from any or all situations, people, events, and so on that
are "holding" you.)

I draw back all these parts of my self into the Wholeness of my Self now.

(Repeat three times or more if needed until you feel strong and centered in the Self. Breathe into your heart center as if the streams of breath
are drawing back these parts into the Wholeness of your Self, centered in
the heart.)

Thank you God, and SO IT IS.

Building a Divine Armor

I now allow my heart to open to God's love.
I now allow the radiant light of God to pour into my being.
I let God's grace fill my energy field with such beauty,
Such light, such wholeness.
I AM filled with the light of God.
I AM now released from psychic bondage.
All psychic ropes that have held me in bondage
Are now lovingly untied and loosed, released, and let go.
All psychic nets that have imprisoned my energy field
Are now dissolved and lifted.
They are released into the nothingness
Of which they truly are.
I now see myself boarding a ship.
The sails are flapping in the wind,
I AM riding far away from the psychic astral realm,
Into the bright sunlight of God's love.
I AM now enclosed in a divine, God-filled bubble.
Of beauteous, iridescent, shimmering light of such radiance.
This God-filled bubble is a golden, multicolored sphere
With white, and luminous purple,
Pink, blue, green, and silver light,
Filling, surrounding, penetrating,
And permeating my energy field.
This beauteous, impenetrable sphere of light
Now protects, seals, and heals me.
I know that any and all seeming
Holes, punctures, and piercings
That have torn my energy field
As a result of my association with any
Person, place, organization,
Situation, circumstance, or addiction
That has influenced me adversely
Are now sealed with the divine energy of the white fire

And the beauteous golden light of unconditional love.
Thank you God, and SO IT IS.

Auric Anomalies

In the last few years, I have noticed some interesting phenomena in auras during healing sessions with clients. Psychic ties have always been visible through clairvoyant sight. But now bizarre anomalies have cropped up, such as psychic nets, plates, armors, hooks, clamps, shackles, jail cells, tentacles, and other strange manifestations. I discovered that human relationships can create unusual configurations in human energy fields.

In the laboratory of Thelma Moss at UCLA in the 1970s, studies showed how the human energy field reacts to emotion. When two people generated enough hostility towards each other, the corona between their fingers abruptly cut off, leaving a gap so sharp and clear, it became known as the "haircut effect." In some instances a bright bar, such as a barrier, appeared between the two photographed fingertips.

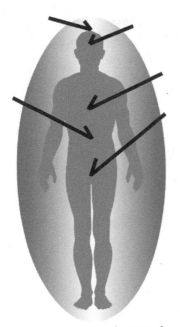

Figure 10c. Psychic Hooks

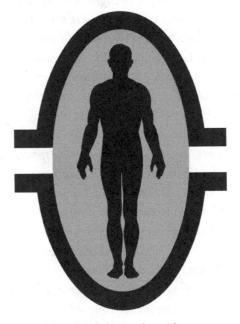

Figure 10d. Psychic Clamps

Further studies involved family groups engaged in family therapy. Group photographs were taken of the fingertips of family members. Typically one member of the group, most often the son, did not photograph at all. Other photographs in this study suggested that high-voltage photography could provide insights into emotional reactions between people.

Your energy field is inextricably connected to the network of energy that covers this entire planet. Humans affect each other in profound ways, and these effects are often deposited into a person's energy field. Some effects, such as love and goodwill, are positive. Others, such as manipulation, control, exploitation, and coercion, are malevolent.

Now you will learn how to heal many of these psychic intrusions that bind you to others in unhealthy ways.

Healing Psychic Bondage

I believe that psychic ties are the most misunderstood anomaly in the human energy field. That is because most people fail to differentiate psychic ties from love ties.

Please refer to Figure 10e on page 168. Psychic ties consist of undue attachments or repulsions to any person, place, thing, organization, circumstance, memory, experience, or addiction that influences you adversely. Psychic ties are built of negative thought-forms and emotions, and they are created without conscious knowledge of their existence. For example, if you have an argument with your boss, what is left over after that argument? A residue of energy that creates a psychic tie.

With clairvoyant sight, psychic ties appear as gray or black (or other color) ropes, cords, strings, webs, dreadlocks, or other nasty, chain-like configurations attached to your energy centers. These shackles of energy are never helpful or beneficial. They serve no one. Therefore, all psychic bonds need to be severed and dissolved.

Please refer to Figure 10f on page 169. In contrast to psychic ties, love ties are true love bonds with all your loved ones, both alive and deceased. These ties also link you to the God of your own personal understanding, your higher self, angels, and inner spiritual teachers. These golden ties of true love can never be broken.

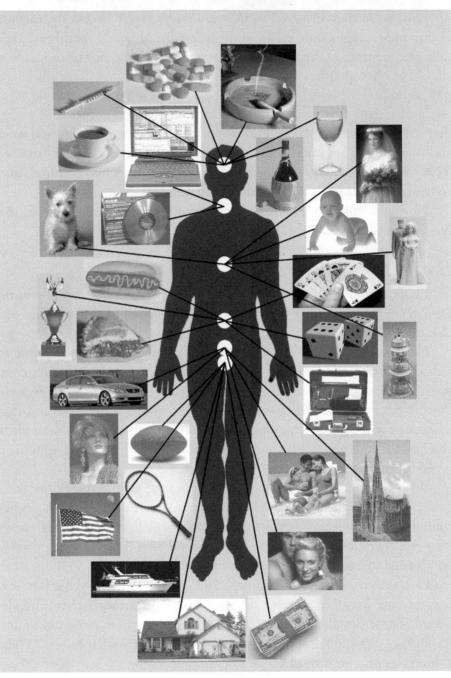

Figure 10e. Psychic Ties

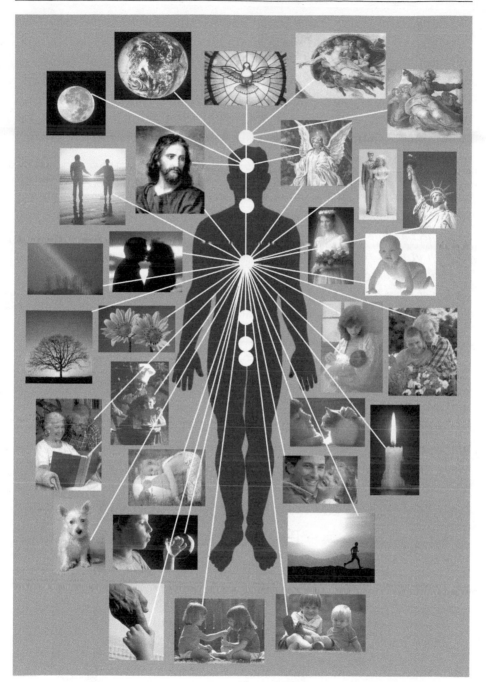

Figure 10f. Love Ties

Because most people mistake psychic ties for love ties, they are reluctant to sever them. However, if you understand that psychic ties deplete your energy field and therefore eventually create disease in your physical body, you will realize how essential it is to cut psychic ties daily with all people in your life. In fact, I guarantee that if you cut psychic ties with all your coworkers in your office and all your loved ones at home on a daily basis, you will have better, more intimate relationships.

Marg Hux from Hamilton, Ontario, Canada, says, *"The ability to truly connect and to feel close with another person is greatly enhanced by cutting psychic ties. It does not mean that I am more "alone," but that I am more able to connect and be close. When I'm not projecting onto the other person my own illusion of what they are supposed to be, I'm more able to see who they are. It is a path of loving with an open hand and heart and constantly giving up my wishes of what will be to allow what is."*

If you have a codependent or addictive relationship with anything or anyone, cutting psychic ties several times a day is crucial. Psychic ties are created every time you have sex, so it is essential to cut psychic ties after every sexual encounter. The umbilical cord attached to your navel from your mother still exists as a psychic tie in adulthood. It is important to cut that tie, especially when your mother dies.

Ira Switzer from San Diego wrote me the following email, *"I was very afraid when I cut ties with my girlfriend that the connection and love [were] being cut, and that I would lose her. It surprised me when I next saw her that the care and common ground was still there. Yet any fear, anxiety, anger was gone, and I was not bugged or fearful of things I had been bothered by before."*

Psychic Tie Cut

(for releasing and dissolving binding ties)
I call upon the Holy Spirit
To cut any and all psychic ties between myself and
(name a person, place, thing, or addiction here).
These psychic ties are now lovingly
Cut, lifted, loved, healed, released, and let go

Into the light of God's love and truth.
Thank you God, and SO IT IS.

Lisa Arlington, a secretary from Chicago, reports, *"My boss was on the warpath for a few weeks since I made a critical mistake. I decided to use Susan's affirmations for cutting psychic ties. The moment I said the prayer, it took the edge off. I felt more relaxed immediately. After saying it a few times over a two-day period, my relationship with my boss changed. He even came into my office and apologized for getting so angry."*

Psychic Tie Cut: Layer by Layer

(for cutting stronger, more impervious ties)
I call upon the Holy Spirit to cut any and all
Astral and psychic ties and karmic bonds between myself and
(name a person, place, thing, or addiction here).
These astral and psychic ties are now
Permanently and completely, lovingly, yet fully
Cut, cut, cut, cut, cut, cut, cut, cut, cut, cut
(repeat until it feels complete)
Lifted, loved, blessed, healed, forgiven, freed,
Released, and completely let go
Layer by layer, by layer, by layer, group by group, by group,
(repeat until it feels complete)
Thank you God, and SO IT IS.

Angela Covello of Morristown, New Jersey, writes, *"I have a close friend with an uncanny telepathic connection to me. One day, as I visually imagined my energy field, I "saw" a silver-gray cord, like an umbilical cord, stretching off into the distance. It was very thick at my solar plexus. About one foot from my body it became the thickness of a large thumb. It was pulsing with life. Although I was at first hesitant, eventually I imagined taking a pair of strong scissors and cut this cord. Then I healed and soothed my energy body where it connected and also sent healing to my friend. The intent and saying the tie-cut prayer certainly is effective. The love between us has increased since cutting the ties."*

As you use psychic tie-cut affirmations, you might also pretend that you are cutting the ties with a light-sword, scissors, or a knife as you repeat, "Cut, cut, cut, cut, cut." Travis Wyly, from England, Arkansas, shares the following experience: "*This morning I began using the prayer for cutting psychic ties to specific individuals in my life. Archangel Michael appeared with a great pair of golden scissors, which he gave me to cut the ties. As I did, tears came to my eyes. Then I saw a mass of energy that represented a specific event from a few years ago. I saw the incredible attachment I had to this event and to its consequences, spanning over a period of years. I saw my energy circuits plugged into this entity. I saw the façade I had created around this event and realized it was time to let it go. The tie or cord to it was massive.*

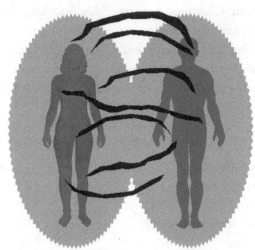

Figure 10g. Heavy Psychic Cords

Suddenly all my inner teachers were present: Michael, Jesus, my Guide and his guide and others in my Soul Group. I took the scissors and began cutting the cord. Tears began to flow. I saw an incredible light that was the center of the Milky Way Galaxy, and as I cut the last remnant of the cord, the mass of whirling energy floated away and was dissolved in the Light. There was rejoicing. Thank you, Father-Mother God."

Healing Psychic Aura Anomalies

If someone attempts to dominate, control, or coerce you, they might deposit psychic ties, bonds, hooks, clamps, plates, and other anomalies into your auric field. These deposits are products of aggression. They are often installed into your energy field consciously and purposefully through energy portals—tubes for traveling into and out of your aura via energy vortices—energy flows going into or out of a portal.

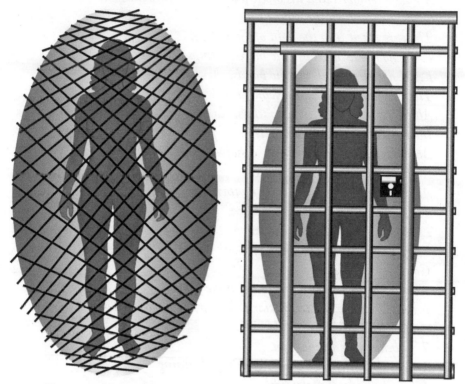

Figure 10h. Psychic Net   *Figure 10i. Psychic jail*

Psychic Anomaly Healing

Use the following prayer to heal any such anomalies:
Any and all psychic nets, fishing nets,
Clamps, shackles, hooks, plates, and jails
That have been installed in my energy field
Are now dissolved and healed with the divine acid,
All these psychic implants are now lovingly
Lifted, lifted, lifted, lifted, lifted, lifted, lifted,
Dissolved, dissolved, healed, and released,

Lifted into the light of God's love and truth.
Any all psychic fishing hooks that were placed in my energy field
Are now removed and dissolved with the divine acid.
They are burnt in the divine fire.
They are lifted into the light of God's love.
I AM now free of all psychic hooks, clamps, and boots.
I AM now free of all psychic bonds,
Ties, shackles, nets, and psychic jails.
All ties, bonds, jails, nets, shackles, clamps,
Boots, hooks, cordings, tentacles, and portals
Are now lovingly cut, severed, dissolved, and destroyed.
And the source and its creators
Are now prevented from creating them again.
These are all now dissolved, healed,
Lifted, released, blessed, and let go.
They are lifted into the light of God's love, God's peace,
God's power, and God's glory.
The beauteous violet flame of Saint Germain
Is now cleansing, clearing, clarifying,
And healing my energy field.
This beauteous divine light
Is now cleansing, cleansing cleansing, cleansing,
Like a tornado of violet fire
Now moving through my energy field.
Cleansing, cleansing, cleansing, cleansing,
Healing, healing, healing, healing,
Lifting, lifting, lifting, lifting.
This beauteous violet divine energy,
This beauteous violet flame tornado,
Cleansing my energy field,
Now continues to cleanse my energy field
Until it is no longer needed.
Thank you God, and SO IT IS.

Healing Psychic Coercion
(for preventing anyone from manipulating, controlling, or coercing you)
I call upon the Holy Spirit to cut any and all psychic ties

Between myself and (insert name of person here).
These psychic ties are now lovingly
Cut, lifted, loved, healed, released, and let go
Into the light of God's love and truth.
I invoke the divine presence
To eliminate all negations and limitations
That no longer serve me.
I now dispel all negations of psychic coercion,
And any other thoughts and emotions
That do not reflect the truth of my being.
They are now lovingly lifted, transmuted, and transformed
Through the power of the Holy Spirit.
I AM now open and free to embrace positive,
Life-supporting, energizing thoughts and emotions.
I now welcome thoughts
Of self-authority and freedom of expression.
I call upon Holy Spirit to release all coercion
And to build a beautiful golden sphere
Of protective divine love and light around me.
I call upon Holy Spirit to give me the will
To follow my own true heart and mind now.
I AM in balance. I AM in control.
I AM the only authority in my life.
I AM divinely protected by the light of my being.
I close off my aura and body of light
To all but my own God-self.
Thank you God, and SO IT IS.

Reversing Black Magic

(for healing dark energies, spells, curses, talismans, totems, and black magic)
Any and all astral entities, thought-forms, implants,
And negative energies that have been deposited
Into my energy field by (insert name of person here)
Through totems or talismans, minerals or gems,
Through words, thoughts, intentions, psychic vampirism,
Circles, spells, enchantments, curses, black magic,
And all other manipulative methods of psychic coercion,

Whether known or unknown, conscious or subconscious,
I know that these entities and negative energies
Are now lovingly healed and forgiven.
You are now lovingly lifted in love.
You are unified with the truth of being.
You are united with God's divine love,
Divine light, and divine truth.
Beloved ones, go now in love, go now in truth.
You are bless-ed, forgiven, and released
Into the love, light, and wholeness of
The universal God Consciousness.
Go in peace now. Go in light. Go in love. Go in peace.
Thank you God, and SO IT IS.

One of my students, Joshua Minquist, complained that he felt he was under the influence of a spell or curse that had been placed on him. After using the previous prayer, Reversing Black Magic, and the next one, Releasing Agreements, he wrote me the following email: *"Thank you, Susan. I am experiencing powerful love and golden energy right now. After breaking bonds, I have now canceled all agreements and forgiven all curses. I now look forward and not back."*

Releasing Agreements[5]

An agreement, contract, or vow with a person, entity, or seeming dark forces can bind your energy field for lifetimes with psychic nets, clamps, and jails. If you become aware that such energies are affecting you or others, then use the following affirmation to eliminate such contracts:

I call upon Jesus Christ, Lord Sananda and Divine Mother
To cancel, release and dissolve
Any contracts, agreements, vows, commitments,
Exchanges, trades or relationships I may have made
At any time in my multidimensional existence,
Which are limiting my Wholeness in any way.
These commitments, vows, contracts, trades,
Exchanges, agreements and relationships
Are now dissolved, released, cancelled, let go,
Made null and void on every level

Of my multidimensional existence,
In the name and through the power of Jesus Christ,
In the name and through power of Lord Sananda,
In the name and through the power of Divine Mother.
I know that I AM free.
All frameworks, structures, circuitry,
And multidimensional matrices
That have developed as a result
Of these now cancelled contracts
Are now dissolved, collapsed, let go,
Released on every level of my energy field now.
And I AM opening fully in Wholeness of Divine Love,
Aligning with Wholeness of Divine Truth,
Allowing Wholeness of Divine Grace.
Thank you God, and SO IT IS.

Shielding From Lower Energies

It is vital not to be overly concerned or paranoid about psychic coercion. There is nothing to fear. There is no "evil" that will "attack" you. There is no "bad" energy "out there." Vampirism is a quality of weakness in others, and that weakness feeds on your light and strength. As you continue to use affirmations and prayers, such as the Self-Authority Affirmation, and as you continue to grow in self-authority, you will stay grounded in Spirit, in the true nature of your being—God Consciousness. You will no longer invite lower energies. Therefore use the following affirmation:

I AM filled with the light of God. My cup runneth over.
The light of God fills and surrounds me now.
I AM so full with the divine presence
That nothing else can penetrate my divine beingness.
I AM full. I AM filled with God's strength,
God's power, God's love, and God's light.
Thank you God, and SO IT IS.

Prayer Before Sleep

The following prayer can be used right before sleep to strengthen your energy field and prevent psychic attack or vampirism during sleep. This simple prayer can avert nightmares, fitful sleep, or broken sleep. You will sleep more soundly and peacefully.

I open my heart to God's love.
I AM a beloved child of God.
I AM filled with the light of God.
I AM a beauteous being of great power,
Great energy, great good and great glory.
I now call upon God
To keep me protected, safe, and secure
In God Consciousness during sleep.
I now call upon God to build a beautiful golden sphere
Of divine love and light around me as I sleep,
To keep me safe, secure, and one with God.
Thank you God, and SO IT IS.

In the next chapter, you practice powerful methods to heal your mental body of negative energies, beliefs, habits, and conditions.

11

Your Mind: Your Worst Enemy?

ဢ

Transforming Your Mental Body

"Lead me from the unreal to the real! Lead me from darkness
to light."

—The Upanishads[1]

Is your mind your worst enemy? Well, it can be an enemy or your best
friend, depending on how you use it. Your mind can be a pristine, joyous
abode of peace, or a flaming habitat of hell. When outer circumstances and
adverse situations weigh heavily on your mind, then your haven of peace
can turn into a nightmare. Yet you have inner power to transform your
mind and return to peace. Prayer is a powerful way to do this.

Your mind is housed in an area of your auric field called the *mental
body*. This body is often seen clairvoyantly with streaks of strong colors
that change and shift according to moods and emotions. In this chapter
you will learn to heal your mental body through the power of prayer and
affirmation.

Healing Your Mental Body

Your mental body is built of thought-forms so intense that they
congeal into solid form. This collection of thoughts determines your

experience in life. In other words, you create your own life based on beliefs, habits, conditions, emotions, and intentions. Because you have free will, you are in charge of what happens to you. In fact, nothing ever happens "to you." You only happen to yourself.

For example, if you continually think or say, "I am fat, I am fat," then that thought is strongly implanted into your mind. And your subconscious mind always says yes to every deeply felt and believed intention. So the manifestation of fatness will occur, just as you have affirmed and pictured it.

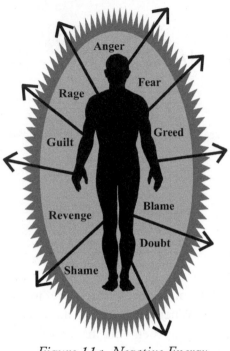

Figure 11a. Negative Energy

Thought-forms affect not only yourself but also others. Have you ever been in an enclosed space with someone whose energy field makes you feel so uncomfortable, agitated, and suffocated that you must leave immediately? Negative thought-forms project that kind of repellent energy. Please refer to Figure 11a. An aura becomes bristly when it is filled with negative thoughts and emotions. A sensitive person who gets near a brittle energy field is repulsed by that energy.

Think of your auric field as a pond. When you drop a rock into the center of the pond, then the waves of water ripple outward in concentric circles until the ripples hit the outer edge. Then these ripples move back to the center of the pond. Similarly, your thought-forms broadcast from your auric field out to the universe. Then they return to you, just as they were transmitted.

Please refer to Figures 11b and 11c on the following page. If your energy field is filled with positive, smooth, stable, joyful, peaceful, tranquil, content, serene, loving thoughts and feelings, then you will magnetize positive experiences. However, if your auric field is poisoned with negative,

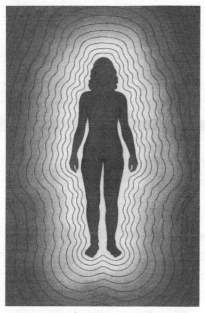
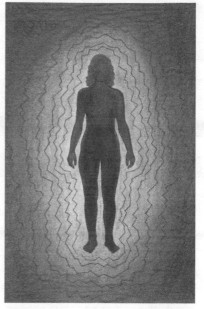

Figure 11b. Positive Thoughts   *Figure 11c. Negative Thoughts*

hateful, angry, vengeful, depressing, chaotic, anxious, irritating, jagged, toxic thoughts and emotions, then you will attract difficult, negative situations.

The mind of the woman in Figure 11c is acting as her enemy. However, she can transform it into her best friend. Using the Thought-Form Healing Prayer can transform your mind from anguish into heavenly paradise in a matter of moments. This prayer can heal anything—any physical, mental, emotional, or other problem in your life. This healing prayer is a way to take control of your thoughts by using a simple formula.

Thought-Form Healing Prayer

As you read the Thought-Form Healing (on page 183) aloud, please close your eyes when you come to the first blank space. Get in touch with what you are feeling. Speak aloud whatever negative emotions and thoughts are coming up for you. Then, when you come to the second blank space, close your eyes again and speak the opposite correlates of the feelings that came up in the first blank space.

Here are a few examples of negative thoughts and their positive correlates. This chart can help you decide what to put in the second blank space.

Negative Thoughts	Positive Correlates
1. Anger	1. Forgiveness
2. Sadness	2. Happiness
3. Guilt	3. Self-Forgiveness
4. Blame	4. Self-Responsibility
5. Depression	5. Inspiration
6. Hatred	6. Love
7. Self-hatred	7. Self-worth
8. Poverty	8. Abundance
9. Fear	9. Courage
10. Resentment	10. Forgiveness
11. Insecurity	11. Confidence
12. Shyness	12. Outgoingness
13. Rejection	13. Self-acceptance
14. Doubt	14. Faith
15. Loss	15. Wholeness
16. Addiction	16. Self-Empowerment
17. Illness	17. Wellness
18. Inflexibility	18. Flexibility
19. Egotism	19. Humility
20. Condemnation	20. Commendation
21. Coercion	21. Permissiveness
22. Disrespect	22. Respect
23. Attachment	23. Letting go
24. Exhaustion	24. Vitality
25. Frustration	26. Nonresistance
27. Agitation	28. Serenity
29. Worry	29. Peacefulness
30. Evasion	30. Responsibility
31. Pressure	31. Resourcefulness
32. Burden	32. Letting go
33. Jealousy	34. Goodwill
34. Perfectionism	34. Self-Love
35. Impatience	35. Patience
36. Error	36. Forgiveness
37. Selfishness	37. Altruism
38. Grief	38. Comfort
39. Confusion	39. Clarity
40. Aging	40. Youthfulness

Now speak the Thought-Form Healing Prayer audibly in a strong, clear voice. All affirmations and prayers in this book are to be spoken with conviction, confidence, and certainty. All of these affirmations can be used to heal yourself or to heal others. When praying for others, simply replace "I" and "me" with the name of the person you are praying for.

Thought-Form Healing Prayer

I invoke the divine presence to eliminate
All negations and limitations that no longer serve me.
I now dispel all negations of (list negative thoughts here)
And any other thoughts and emotions
That do not reflect the truth of my being.
They are now lovingly lifted, transmuted, and transformed
Through the power of the Holy Spirit.
I AM now open and free to embrace positive,
Life-supporting, energizing thoughts and emotions.
I now welcome thoughts of (list positive correlates here).
I AM in balance. I AM in control.
Thank you God, and SO IT IS.

Universal Thought-Form, Pattern, and Belief-Structure Healing

The following prayer can be used whenever negative thoughts and feelings are so overwhelming that they seem to dominate you. No habit, belief, or thought can control you when you use the power of prayer to heal it. As you read this aloud, close your eyes when you come to the first blank space. Speak audibly whatever negative feelings and thoughts are coming up for you. When you come to the second blank space, again close your eyes and speak the opposite correlates of the feelings that came up in the first blank space.

I now call forth the Holy Spirit,
The spirit of wholeness, love, and truth,
To illuminate the truth upon any and all erroneous
Thought-forms, thought-patterns, and thought-structures
That obscure the truth in this situation now.
Through the healing divine light of the Holy Spirit,
I dissolve any and all negative thought-forms,

Structures, patterns, and belief systems.
This light of truth is completely permeating
And suffusing all negativity in this situation, place,
And states of consciousness related to it.
I know that any and all limiting thought-forms,
Thought-patterns, thought-concepts, and thought-structures
Are now easily and effortlessly dissolved
By the healing divine light of truth
Of the Holy Spirit, and the law of first cause,
Into the nothingness of what they truly are.
The Holy Spirit now suffuses, shines upon, lifts,
And transmutes any and all thought-forms of
(list negative thoughts here).
These negative thought-forms, thought-structures, and thought-concepts
Are now lovingly and permanently lifted, healed,
Released, let go, and transmuted into the good,
And they are gone. (Take a deep breath to release.)
Through the purifying power of the Holy Spirit,
They are now blessed, transformed, and transfigured.
Into their divine true archetypes of
(list positive correlates here).
I AM in control of my mind. I AM empowered now,
Through the light of the Holy Spirit
With the healing, purifying, and sanctifying power
Of the Holy Spirit and the God Consciousness within me.
I AM divinely protected and guided into uplifted, true,
More powerfully God conscious living and being
Right here and right now.
Thank you God, and SO IT IS.

Rakshasas Healing Prayer

Rakshasas, mentioned in the ancient scriptures of India, are demonic thought-forms built of such intense energies that they take on a life of their own. Examples of rakshasas are entities placed in mechanical objects by people who curse their cars, washing machines, computers, and so forth. Devils, Satan, Lucifer, and other imaginary demonic entities are given life by intensely concentrated collective beliefs and thought-forms. Here is a prayer to heal rakshasas:

I now know that any and all demonic energies,
Thought-forms, and rakshasas, are now
Lovingly healed and forgiven. You are lifted in divine love.
You are dissolved, healed, released, and let go
Into the nothingness of what you truly are.
You have no power over me.
You have no control over my life.
You are now commanded
To release the hold that you have had over me.
You can no longer take control of me or of my life.
You are now commanded to go into the divine light now.
Go with God now and dissolve into nothingness.
Go now, in peace and love.
Thank you God, and SO IT IS.

Healing Past Experiences

Your energy field carries a burden of experiences and memories from your past—from this life and from previous lives. These are stored in your subconscious mental body, just as a computer hard drive stores data. In this section you will let go of the past so your energy field can be free of the weight of past yokes of false responsibility, guilt, blame, and resentment.

Past Experience Healing

All experiences, core, record, memory, and effects
Are transmuted and transformed into pure love and light
By the violet flame of limitless transmutation.
I have a clean blank slate on which to write new experiences.
I AM transformed by the renewing of my mind, right now.
I close all doors, openings, and holes to my past now.
I AM vibrating at such a high frequency of love,
That I AM free from all
Past burdens and false responsibilities.
I AM a God/Goddess of great love, light, and glory.
Thank you God, and SO IT IS.

Letting Go Prayer

When you hold on to the past, your energy field is cluttered with dark, deep-seated, entrenched energies. Letting go of these vibrations lifts your aura into a higher, more refined frequency. This prayer will help.

I let go of worn-out things, hopeless conditions,
Useless ideas, and futile relationships now.
Divine right order and divine right timing
Are now established and maintained
In my mind, body, relationships, finances,
In all of my affairs, and in my world,
Through the power of the Holy Spirit
And my own indwelling God Consciousness now.
Divine circulation is at work in my life,
And the inflow and outflow
Of everything in my life is in divine order.
I AM peaceful, balanced, and poised.
This is so now, in God's own wise and perfect ways.
Thank you God, and SO IT IS.

Forgiveness Prayer

An unforgiving energy field is mired with psychic ties, nets, and other shadowy anomalies that bind you to past trauma, hate, and resentment. True forgiveness of yourself, of others, and of life situations dissolves binding ties and lifts your energy field more quickly than just about anything else. Forgiveness places the situation under the law of grace. It is an ongoing, lifelong project of highest importance. No life can be happy or completely fulfilled without true forgiveness.

Use the following forgiveness prayer up to 30 minutes per day to supercharge your spiritual growth. However, most people find it so powerful that five minutes per day is suggested as the recommended amount.

By and through the power of the Holy Spirit,
I know and decree right now
That all that has seemingly offended me or held me,
I now forgive and release.
Within and without, I now forgive and release.

Things past, things present, and all things future,
I now forgive and release.
I forgive and release everything and everyone everywhere
Who can possibly need forgiveness or release.
This includes forgiveness for myself
Through the power of God now.
I forgive and I release absolutely everyone and everything,
Past, present, and future.
Everything and everyone from my past, present, and future
That could possibly need to forgive and release me,
Including myself, does so now.
This is done now by and through the power of God,
The God Consciousness in me, and within us all.
I AM free and all others concerned are now free also.
Therefore all things are completely cleared up among us all,
Now and forevermore, under grace,
In God's own wise and perfect ways.
Thank you God, and SO IT IS.

Forgiveness Healing Chant

This healing affirmation can forgive any particular person, group, or situation. Use this affirmation for as long as needed, until it feels complete. You can work on a particular relationship, such as a parent, spouse, child, or situation, for as long as you feel guided. With some relationships with lifelong difficulties, you might feel the need to use this for a year or more:

The God Consciousness in me
Is my forgiving and releasing power.
The God Consciousness in (insert name of person here)
Is his/her forgiving and releasing power.
The God Consciousness in me
Is my forgiving and releasing power.
The God Consciousness in (insert name of person here)
Is his/her forgiving and releasing power.
I AM free and he/she is free also.
Therefore, all things are cleared up between us,

Now and forever, under grace, in perfect ways.
Thank you God, and SO IT IS.

Façade Body Healing

A façade body is a set of beliefs held so strongly that they build an armor, mask, or façade in the energy field. Self-absorbed people have murky auras with a thick belt or armor that surrounds their field. Such an aura shuts out love vibrations, disallowing love from flowing in or out. In this case the individual can feel neither loved nor loving. Even a mother's pure,

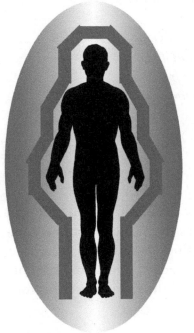

unconditional love can be blocked by such a defensive shield. Feelings are suppressed. Kind thoughts and wishes are obstructed. The auric field might even manifest anomalies, such as a prison or cage.

Before using the following prayer, decide what set of beliefs you want to heal. For example, you might be wearing a façade body of poverty, unworthiness, superiority, inferiority, machismo, timidity, fatness, defensiveness, bullishness, anger, or another mask. Choose one of your façade bodies and call it by name, such as "victim," "self-righteousness," "self-hatred," or any other name that describes it. Then place that name into the appropriate blank spaces in the prayer.

Figure 11d. The Façade Body

Façade Body Healing Prayer

I call upon Holy Spirit
To lovingly shine the light of truth and love
Upon any and all façade bodies of
(insert name of façade body here)
Within myself now. These façade bodies of
(insert name of façade body here)

That are surrounding me
Are now lovingly cracked open, crumbled up,
Dissolved, healed, released,
And let go by the Holy Spirit and
(name of your diety)
Into the light of God's love and truth.
I now call upon my own soul,
My Christ-self and "I AM" self
To fill this space and fill me
With my true divine pattern and soul expression.
Let God's will be done in this matter.
Thank you God, and SO IT IS.

Past Life Mental Body Healing

Your past lives have control over you to the extent that you let them. You can heal past experiences, no matter how traumatic they may be. Remnants of a past life can manifest in your aura as a mental body. Clairvoyants sometimes see a former life face or body in your aura or superimposed on your face or body.

When a person states opinions that reflect prejudices or strong beliefs from a former life, a figure of that past life body may appear in the energy field, dressed in garments of that former life. When the conversation changes, the figure vanishes from the aura.[2] Similarly, when prejudices or strong beliefs learned in childhood are expressed, a parent may hover over the shoulder in the aura. Here is a prayer to heal these mental bodies:

Past Life Mental Body Healing Prayer

I now know that any and all past life mental bodies
That have influenced me adversely
Are now lovingly lifted in the light of God's love.
You are filled with the light of God's truth.
You are forgiven of any and all
Seeming guilt, shame, confusion, and fear.
You are released of the past and can now move on.
You no longer have any binding influence upon me.
I now release any and all ties and cords

That have bound me to past lives.
They are blessed, lifted, cut, dissolved,
Released, and let go now.
All past life mental bodies are now
Free to move into God's light now.
Go now, in peace and love.
Thank you God, and SO IT IS.

Healing Astral Shells

This last healing prayer is an advanced method of deep spiritual surgery. It heals and lifts severe thought-patterns, structures, and habits that have encased your being in *astral shells*—complex, multilayered, multidimensional belief structures built on façades, constructs, and conditions that have persisted for lifetimes. These shells block spiritual and material progress. Yet, they can be healed through this profound prayer.

Before you begin this prayer, know in your consciousness that no job is too big or too small for the Holy Spirit. In consciousness, address the Holy Spirit concerning healing the entirety of the astral shells that you are dealing with, and the thought-worlds enclosed within them. Read my book *Ascension* to learn about the ascended masters and archangels that are invoked in this prayer.

The Holy Spirit now shines the light of truth upon all these astral shells, thought-forms, supporting thought-structures, and belief systems, all the thought-worlds within them, and upon everything and everyone here concerned. I know this is true multi-dimensionally, multi-temporally, and otherwise, throughout this entire healing process.

The Holy Spirit is infinitely large and infinitely small. I know that no job is too big or too small for the Holy Spirit. I decree the perfect healing of these astral shells, thought-forms, supporting thought-structures, and belief systems, now. This is so, under grace, in God's own wise and perfect ways.

I call upon the Holy Spirit, the Spirit of truth and wholeness, to permeate with the light of truth and wholeness any and all astral shells, thought-forms, supporting thought-structures, and belief systems influencing (insert name of person here), *that are wise to heal, and need healing now. I know and decree these astral shells, thought-forms, supporting thought-structures, and belief systems, are merely distorted structures of thought. Their size, depth, strength, or length of duration are as nothing before the healing power of the Holy Spirit, Jesus, and the God Consciousness.*

These astral shells, thought-forms, supporting thought-structures, and belief systems are rendered powerless, null, and void, by the power of the Holy Spirit, Jesus, and the God Consciousness, right here and right now. I know all those involved in this healing, both the healed and the healer, are unified with the universal divine mind. We are unified with the mighty I AM divine presence, and the violet flame of ascended divine master Saint Germain. We are one with the transcendent loving wholeness of the Brahman divine consciousness. We are unified with the mighty I AM divine presence within, right here and right now. We are one with the full dimensional wholeness of the God Consciousness, under grace in perfect ways.

I know and decree these astral shells, thought-forms, supporting thought-structures, and belief systems are now lovingly and completely, thoroughly and gently, lifted, healed, forgiven, and released. They are filled and surrounded by the golden, yellow, silver, and white, archangelic and sacred fire and light of the Holy Spirit, Archangel Christ Michael and the divine archangels, under grace in perfect ways.

These astral shells, thought-forms, supporting thought-structures, and belief systems are completely healed now. They are lovingly burnt up in the sacred fire. They are filled with this holy light. They are lifted and transmuted by the golden, yellow, silver, and white, archangelic, and sacred fire and light of the Holy Spirit, and archangels of the Seven Rays: Archangel Christ Michael, Archangel Christ Gabriel, Archangel Christ Raphael, Archangel Christ Chamuel, Archangel Christ Zadkiel, Archangel Christ Uriel, and Archangel Christ Jophiel.

They are lovingly lifted and transformed by the full wholeness, light, and healing of these archangels of the seven rays. They are lovingly lifted and transformed by the full wholeness, light, and healing of the presence of the almighty Father-Mother God, Jesus, and the Holy Spirit, under grace in perfect ways.

These astral shells, thought-forms, supporting thought-structures, and belief systems are lovingly lifted, blessed, healed, forgiven, and released.

They are lifted, healed, forgiven, and released by the golden, yellow, sil-
ver, and white archangelic and sacred fire and light of the Holy Spirit
and the divine archangels of the seven rays. I know the God Conscious-
ness, in full harmony and cooperation with all the angelic and arch-
angelic hosts, completes this healing now. I decree these astral shells,
thought-forms, and supporting thought-structures to be fully healed
now, under grace in God's own wise and perfect ways. Thank you God,
and SO IT IS.

Next, do any additional healing that comes up because of healing these shells.

This prayer, and several other prayers in the last three chapters, were developed by my beloved teacher Rich Bell, who is no longer in embodiment. For more information about using healing prayers, read and study my books *Miracle Prayer, Instant Healing, Divine Revelation,* and *How to Hear the Voice of God,* and take classes or sessions. Teachers are listed at *www.divinerevelation.org/Teachers.html.* Or order a home study course at *www.divinerevelation.org.*

In the next chapter, you will learn more profound prayers that energize, strengthen, lift, and fill your energy field with divine light, love, truth, and grace.

12

The Healing Power of Prayer

ꙁꙁ

Purifying Your Auric Field

"It only takes a little light to dispel much darkness."

—Anonymous[1]

Consistent contact with God's transforming tools, which lift you into conscious union with God, allows you to heal any condition. These tools are Divine Love, Divine Light, Divine Truth, and Divine Grace. The prayers here dissolve fear, pain and depression from your energy field by placing you in the vibration of divine love. Reciting these powerful, energizing prayers lifts the frequency of your aura dramatically.

To practice these prayers, center in your heart. Breathe into the heart and begin saying the prayers audibly in a normal speaking voice. Or you can record them onto an audiotape or CD and then sit comfortably, close your eyes, relax, and playback the audio recording to use as a guided meditation.

These prayers are written by Connie Huebner, founder of Divine Mother's Vibrational Tools, a methodology for opening you to God's unmanifest wholeness.

Divine Light Prayer[2]

Divine Light is pouring into me now. Divine Light is filling my energy field on every level, from most dense to most etheric, akashic and every place in between, multi-dimensionally, multi-temporally and otherwise. Divine Light is opening within me now. I AM receiving more and more Divine Light, moment by moment. Divine Light is healing every limitation within my energy system and opening me to Wholeness now. Divine Light is releasing all energies of discord and opening my awareness to Divine Truth, so that more Divine Light can flood my energy system now.

I accept Divine Light within me now and I know that Divine Light is increasing its presence within my system and illuminating my entire energy field. The most rare, delicate quality of light in creation is opening in my energy system and lifting my energy field into resonance with Sacred Light vibration.

Sacred Light vibration is creating Wholeness within my multidimensional energy system now. Sacred Light vibration is opening, lifting, cleansing, and freeing my entire energy system now, and Sacred Light vibration is allowing my energy system to know Truth. Sacred Light vibration is increasing its presence within my energy system. Divine Light is filling me now and opening me to more light.

I AM lifted, opened, cleansed, and freed in Divine Light. (You can repeat this phrase several times if you like.)

Divine Light is emerging from Source and overflowing on every level of my energy field until there is nothing left but Divine Light holding my multidimensional energy system and feeding my multidimensional energy system.

I AM filled with Light.

I open to more Light.

I know Sacred Light.

I allow Sacred Light to resonate fully throughout my multidimensional energy system now, and fill me with Divine Light.

I AM Divine Light now, multi-dimensionally and otherwise.

I live in Divine Light and increase Divine Light again and again.

Thank you God, and SO IT IS.

Divine Truth Prayer[3]

Divine Truth is opening in Wholeness within my energy system now. Divine Truth knows only Truth and is resonating Truth throughout my energy system, releasing all untruth. Divine Truth knows Wholeness and fills me with the Wholeness of Divine Truth. All untruth anywhere in my multi-dimensional energy system is releasing, letting go, opening in Truth. Divine Truth is Whole and complete within my energy system and heals me in Truth. Truth knows Wholeness and allows Wholeness to be fully present within my energy system.

Divine Truth knows me intimately and fills me with Truth. Truth is opening in Wholeness again and again throughout my energy system, freeing me from all untruth on every level in every place and point of my energy field. I AM healing in Wholeness of Divine Truth. I am Wholeness of Divine Truth.

Thank you God, and SO IT IS.

Divine Love Prayer[4]

Wholeness of Divine Love is pouring into my energy field now. The lively, radiant presence of Divine Love is filling my energy field now. The radiant presence of Divine Love is moving everywhere within my energy system. Divine Love is saturating my energy field. Divine Love is increasing and intensifying its presence moment by moment within my energy field now. The lively, dynamic energy of Divine Love is clearing, opening and transmuting all energies of lack and limitation within my energy system, multi-dimensionally, multi-temporally, and otherwise. My system is opening to the presence of more and more life energy of Divine Love. The vital life energy of Divine Love is transmuting all energies of discord and limitation within my system now. Radiant, vibrant Divine Love is transmuting all error conditioning, all error patterning, all limited belief systems and all limiting self-concepts.

Divine Love is radiant within my energy field. Divine Love is increasing its presence within my energy field. The life energy of Divine Love is pulsating within my energy system now, in complete unison with the heartbeat of the Creator. My energy system is radiant with Divine Love.

The dynamic pulsations of Divine Love within my energy system are clearing and transmuting all limitation and discord in my system now. I AM one with the fullness of God's Love.

Thank you God, and SO IT IS.

Ascending Light Prayer[5]

Ascending Light vibration is entering my energy system now. Ascending Light vibration is moving into every level of my multidimensional energy system. Ascending Light vibration is filling my energy system. Ascending Light is resonating on every level of my system, opening it to more Ascending Light.

Ascending Light vibration is lifting and clearing all ancestral patterning within my energy system. Ascending Light vibration is freeing my system from all limiting energies and frequencies. Ascending Light vibration is filling my entire energy system, lifting me into Ascending Light. Every level of my system is receiving Ascending Light. I AM radiant with Ascending Light, and Ascending Light is increasing its presence within my energy system moment by moment.

My limited DNA patterning is releasing in Ascending Light vibration. Ascending Light vibration is filling my DNA system, releasing old limiting patterning and filling my DNA system with Ascending Light. Ascending Light is vibrating throughout my entire energy system—healing, lifting, clearing, opening me to more Ascending Light.

More and more Ascending Light is pouring into my energy system. My energy system is vibrating in Ascending Light, is lifting into Ascending Light. My multidimensional energy system knows Ascending Light. Every molecule, cell, atom, particle, place, and space in my multidimensional system is receiving Ascending Light. My system is opening in Ascending Light again and again as I lift into Ascending Light.

Thank you God, and SO IT IS.

Divine Grace Prayer[6]

I know that the Wholeness of Divine Grace is completely filling my energy field now. Divine Grace is pouring into my energy field now, filling every place in my multidimensional and multi-temporal and otherwise energy system with the presence of Divine Grace. Divine Grace is opening within my energy field on every level from most dense to most etheric, akashic and beyond, and every place in between.

Divine Grace is permeating, penetrating, saturating my energy field with the holy presence of Divine Grace. Divine Grace is opening within every atom, cell, molecule, particle, place, and space within my entire energy system now, more and more wholeness of Divine Grace filling me now. Divine Grace is opening, clearing, balancing, lifting, healing, freeing—holding me in Divine Grace now. More and more wholeness of Divine Grace, wholeness is pouring into wholeness, pouring into more wholeness of Divine Grace.

I AM lifted, opened, cleansed, and freed in the wholeness of Divine Grace (repeat until clear). *This is occurring now under Grace in God's most wise and perfect ways.*

Thank you God, and SO IT IS.

Rev. Connie Huebner is the founder of Divine Mother's Vibrational Tools and the Divine Mother Church. She has a BA from the University of North Carolina, Chapel Hill, and a master's degree in Research in Consciousness from Maharishi European Research University. She has been a Transcendental Meditation teacher for 30 years. For more information about Divine Mother's Vibrational Tools, go to *www.divinemotheronline.net*.[7]

Connie Huebner is one of the recommended teachers listed on my Website at *www.divinerevelation.org/Teachers.html*.

In the next chapter, you will use profound vibrations of color and sound to augment and strengthen your auric field.

Part IV

୨୦

Strengthening Your Energy Field

13

Using Color and Sound

ॐ

Lifting Vibrational Energy

"There is no darkness if you face the sun."

—Amar Jyoti[1]

In India and China, color and sound therapy have healed people for millennia. In healing temples of ancient Egypt, rooms of specific shapes and colors enhanced therapeutic vibrations. In 500 BC, Pythagoras, a Greek philosopher, used color and music therapy to treat patients. Mantras, prayers, or seed sounds that produce harmonious, healing vibrations are chanted in many religious traditions.

Because your subtle energy field is made of vibration and light, it is most profoundly transformed through light or sound. This chapter will introduce color and sound therapies as energy-enhancing measures.

Reactions to Color

Do your favorite colors brighten your day? Are you attracted to certain colors and repelled by others? You probably choose favorite colors for clothing and home décor. This is because unique vibratory frequencies radiate from different colors, forming patterns that collide either positively or negatively with your energy field.

The colors and energy in your aura are determined not only by your thoughts and emotions, but also by the light and colors around you. Color starvation can result in disease, disharmony, and even death. People locked in dark rooms for extended periods become weak and ill. By bathing in specific color vibrations, you can increase strength and health. If your color balance tips too much onto one end of the spectrum, basking in colors of the opposite frequency can bring harmony.

Colors have inherent properties and affect you in three basic ways: warming, neutral, and cooling. Red, orange, and yellow are warm, stimulating colors that move toward you and appear bigger. Light colors also appear closer and bigger. That is why traffic signs are yellow or red. Green is a neutral color. Blue, indigo, and violet are cool, calming colors that move away and appear smaller. Dark colors also seem farther away and smaller.

To create a restful, peaceful atmospheric energy, use cool colors. Sunny rooms with southern exposure can be toned down with such colors. To create excitement or cheerfulness, use warm colors. Rooms with northern exposure can be warmed up by such a color palette.

Inharmonious color schemes or overly intense colors in décor or clothing can exhaust and overwhelm your energy field. To reduce intensity and make a color grayer, add its complimentary color, its direct opposite on the color wheel (see Figure 8b on page 126). Or add white, which increases value and decreases intensity. Black reduces value and intensity. Rough surfaces decrease color intensity, while shiny surfaces increase it.

How Colors Can Heal You

In the mid-20th century, a judge in America demanded that his courtroom be painted light, bright, cheerful colors. To him, brightness led to right thinking, and darkness to crooked thinking. Therefore, his court must invoke uplifting feelings. He believed that sitting in a dark, dismal courtroom, day after day, would turn anyone into a criminal. He stated, "White, cream, light yellow, and orange are the colors which are the sanest. I might add light green, for that is the predominant color in nature; black, brown, and deep red are incentives to crime—a man in anger sees red."[2]

Color	Polarity	Effects	Properties
Red	Yang: Male	Stimulates, Vitalizes, Warms, Dilates, Increases Body Heat	Alkaline, Non-electric, Magnetic
Orange	Yang: Male		
Yellow	Yang: Male		
Green	Neutral: Neuter	Balances, Heals, Integrates, Soothes	Neutral
Blue	Yin: Female	Restricts, Slows, Cools, Contracts, Lowers Body Heat	Acidic, Electric, Non-magnetic, Astringent
Indigo	Yin: Female		
Violet	Yin: Female		

The colors of your foods, sunglasses, clothing, home décor, and office décor have profound effects. Blue, indigo, and violet make you introverted and contemplative. Red, orange, and yellow make you energetic and outgoing. Continually absorbing red into your system causes restlessness, irritability, and violence. Too much indigo restricts blood flow and raises blood pressure.

Warm colors stimulate blood flow and remove mucous and toxins. Warm colors increase *anabolism*, or constructive metabolism, by which food is changed into tissue. Cool colors restrict and contract blood vessels. Cool colors increase *catabolism*, or destructive metabolism, by which tissue is broken down into waste products.

In the center of the spectrum, green is totally balanced, with neither a stimulating nor tranquilizing effect.

Wearing Color Vibrations

This table shows correspondences between colors, weekdays, and gemstones. Wearing the color or gemstone of the day can increase that color's vibrational affect on your energy field. Choosing your clothing based on days of the week offers an opportunity to balance your wardrobe with every rainbow color. By wearing all colors of the spectrum each week, you enhance your field with a wide variety of positive energies.

Color:	Red	Orange	Yellow	Green	Blue	Indigo	Violet
Planet:	Sun	Moon	Mars	Mercury	Jupiter	Venus	Saturn
Day of Week:	Sunday	Monday	Tuesday	Wednesday	Thursday	Friday	Saturday
Gem:	Ruby, Red Garnet	Pearl, Moonstone	Red Coral	Emerald, Peridot	Yellow Topaz, Yellow Sapphire	Diamond, Zircon	Blue Sapphire, Blue Topaz, Amethyst

When you wear a gem, have it set in such a way that it touches your skin. In addition, you can prepare a healing solution by soaking a gemstone in water, alcohol, or oil for seven days while the gemstone's energy seeps into the medium. One drop of the solution in a glass of water can be an effective gemstone treatment.

Charging Water With Color

You can charge water with color vibrations by using filters. Fill a glass of water with pure spring water. Then place a transparent colored filter around or on top of the glass. (Order filters at *www.rosco.com/filters*.) Or use a colored glass. Leave the glass of water in sunlight for at least one hour. Store the color-vibration-saturated water in the refrigerator. One or two tablespoons are sufficient for color treatment. Change red, orange, or yellow water every two days in hot weather and every 10 to 14 days in cold weather. Blue, indigo, or violet water stays fresh for seven to 10 days.

Colored Filters

Radiant color is more potent than reflected color. Colored lights, lamps, and sunlight are powerful ways to soak up color vibrations. Ordinary light bulbs are effective light sources to shine through transparent colored filters. Direct sunlight is even more beneficial. A high-tech alternative is a computer and projector, or a large computer screen, with a flat color placed on a PowerPoint slide or on the desktop. Or simply obtain colored light bulbs or colored lampshades. Experiment with these methods to increase a particular color in your energy field.

Treating disease with colored light is a subtle, potent science that requires years of study and experience. Some excellent study guides are available. Refer to Darius Dinshah's *Let There Be Light—Practical Manual for Spectro-Chrome Therapy* and *www.dinshahhealth.org.*

Food-Prana

Color vibrations are imbibed daily through food. Your food color palette is made of pure white sunlight absorbed by plants and animals via photosynthesis. Foods emit particular color vibrations used for growth and vitality. The healthiest diet is a balance of all colors. If your diet is color-deficient, you may suffer color starvation, leading to disease. Often deficiency in particular color vibrations triggers overeating to compensate.

On the following page is a table of common foods and their color vibration. Sometimes the physical color does not correspond with its vibrational color. For example, potatoes vibrate with blue energy, prunes are of yellow vibration, and brown rice vibrates red. No white foods, such as white sugar, white flour, or white rice, are listed here, because they have no color nutritional value.

Red foods activate the liver and produce red blood cells. Yellow fruits and vegetables are laxatives. Orange foods relieve muscle spasms and cramps. Blue foods are cooling, astringent, and antiseptic. Violet destroys worn blood cells and kills harmful bacteria. Green foods are body mineralizers, which regulate metabolism and balance the liver and spleen.

Fresh, organically grown foods instill the greatest pranic power. The longer food is chewed, the more food-prana is imbibed, and the more energy reserves are replenished. When food is not masticated until liquefied, then the full benefits of food-prana are not enjoyed, and the body suffers imperfect digestion. As long as taste still remains in any food particle, nutrition and pranic energy can still be absorbed from it.

COLOR	FOOD			
RED	Cherry	Red Pepper	Red Potato	Pecans
	Red Currant	Red Grape	Whole Wheat	Red Meat
	Red Plum	Tomato	Brown Rice	Liver
	Apple	Watercress	Watermelon	Red Spices
	Strawberry	Spinach	Red Onion	Red Lentil
	Radish	Rhubarb	Red Wine	Raspberry
ORANGE	Peach	Papaya	Sweet Potato	Peanuts
	Tangerine	Apricot	Carrot	Eggs
	Cantaloupe	Orange	Rutabaga	Orange Spices
	Mango	Tangerine	Acorn Squash	Dairy Products
	Persimmon	Pumpkin	Butternut Squash	Gooseberry
YELLOW	Corn	Spaghetti Squash	Grapefruit	Almonds
	Yellow Pepper	Garlic	Honeydew	Cashews
	Yam	White Onion	Prune	Egg Yolk
	Parsnip	Yellow Apple	Fig	Yellow Cheese
	Turnip	Lemon	Bean	White Wine
	Jicama	Banana	Soybean	Poultry
	Yellow Squash	Pineapple	Butter	Yellow Spices
GREEN	Broccoli	Kale	Green Beans	Avocado
	Cauliflower	Bok Choy	Pea	Lime
	Cabbage	Parsley	Sweet Peas	Kiwi
	Brussels Sprouts	Celery	Romaine	Green Pepper
	Swiss Chard	Sprouts, Grasses	Spring Greens	Green Grape
	Turnip Greens	Cucumber	Asparagus	Green Herbs
	Mustard Greens	Fennel	Zucchini Squash	Leek
BLUE	Blueberry	Blue Plum	Potato	Veal
	Bilberry	Black Grape	Raisin	Fish
VIOLET	Pomegranate	Purple Grape	Red Cabbage	Beet
	Cranberry	Purple Broccoli	Eggplant	Beet Tops
	Blackberry	Black Currant		

Red Vibrations

Red, the essence of fire and movement, is a powerful stimulant. Within a few hours of treatment with invigorating red light, patients with depression found relief. Patients with no appetite, when placed in a red chamber, developed a healthy appetite.[3] Red mixed with white, which makes pink, is an antidote that kindles hope for those who suffer from melancholy. However, absorbing too much red causes restlessness and irritability. The phrase "I am seeing red" implies rage and hostility.

INCREASES	Heat, Warmth, Fire, Movement, Vitality, Energy, Stimulation, Excitement, Arousal, Animation, Power, Motivation, Activity, Extroversion, Passion, Sales Success
AGGRAVATES	Overstimulation, Emotions, Rage, Anger, Hostility, Vengeance, Aggression, War, Restlessness, Haste, Agitation, Passion, Lust, Accidents, Fitful Sleep, Insomnia, Rushed Eating, Indigestion
HEALS	Chills, Colds, Influenza, Sluggishness, Tiredness, Inertia, Chronic Fatigue, Congestion, Mucous, Depression, Fear, Timidity, Melancholy, Introversion, Escapism
STIMULATES	Mind, Emotions, Nervous System, Sympathetic Nerves, Circulatory System, Cerebrospinal Fluid, Liver, Appetite, Red Corpuscles, Hemoglobin, Iron Production, Blood Oxygen
SUITABLE FOR	Athletics, Workouts, Weightlifting, Athletic Club Decor, Gymnasium Decor, Store Decor, Restaurant Decor, Sales Attire, Grounding, Taking Action, Motivating People

Orange Vibrations

Orange augments physical and mental vigor, courage, and optimism. It helps "true believers" (those who are gullible, susceptible, or easily taken in by swindlers) gain discrimination. Treatment with orange light increases sensitivity and respect for others. Often called the social color, it increases compassion and overcomes social anxiety. However, too much orange aggravates social superficiality. As a combination of red and yellow, orange increases both physical and mental vigor. Since it is the wisdom ray, orange stimulates creative ideas.

INCREASES	Joyfulness, Optimism, Courage, Physical Energy, Mental Energy, Inner Strength, Mental Clarity, Discernment, Friendliness, Compassion, Social Skills, Respect for Others, Creative Ideas, Artistic Creativity
AGGRAVATES	Overindulgence, Superficiality, Pleasure-Seeking, Codependency, Overeating, Social Butterfies
HEALS	Digestion, Cramps, Muscle Spasms, Osteoporosis, Intestinal Gas, Lungs, Respiratory System, Vocal System, Clinging to Past, Habit Patterns, Conditioning, Prejudice, Cruelty, Critical Tendency, Destructive Tendency, Mistrust, Insecurity, Suspicion, Social Anxiety
STIMULATES	Bone Growth, Circulation, Assimilation, Distribution, Appetite, Nerves, Sexual Energy
SUITABLE FOR	Business Ideas, Creative Think-Tanks, Library Decor, Educational, Buildings, Art Studios, Hospital Decor, Intensive Care, Surgery Prep, Living Rooms, Social Life, Entertainment, Social Decor, Convention Centers, Theaters

Yellow Vibrations

Seeing a bright, golden sunrise or sunset is exulting. Yellow is the essence of luminosity—elevating and joyful. This color stimulates intellectual development and mental power. Mentally challenged children learn more effectively in yellow classrooms.[4] Wearing yellow uplifts your spirit and melts fearful emotions. However, too much yellow can cause arrogance or callousness. The yellow ray rebuilds nerves and releases tension. It can effectively treat paralysis and other nervous disorders. Yellow purifies your body by healing and regulating your organs of elimination. It overcomes constipation and parasites.

INCREASES	Mobility, Activity, Stimulation, Intelligence, Joyfulness, Inspiration, Upliftment, Happiness, Enthusiasm
AGGRAVATES	Acute Inflammation, Fever, Delerium, Diarrhea, Overexcitement, Sleeplessness, Heart Palpitations, Arrogance, Criticism, Robotic Tendencies, Lack of Feeling
HEALS	Constipation, Parasites, Paralysis, Nervous Disorders, Mental Exhaustion, Tension, Depression, Fear, Shame, Treachery, Aversion, Anger, Frustration, Tension, Jealousy, Ignorance, Desire, Worldliness, Avarice, Despondency, Despair, Timidity, Indecisiveness
STIMULATES	Motor Nerves, Building Nerves, Liver, Intestines, Lymph System, Skin, Elimination, Laxative Action, Enzyme Production, Bile Production, Intellect
SUITABLE FOR	Study Rooms, Library Decor, Education, Classroom Decor, Art Studio Decor, Computer Rooms, Office Decor, Bookstore Decor, Bathroom Decor

Green Vibrations

Nature has decked herself in the most soothing color of the rainbow—green. Clear, springtime, bright grass-green colors stimulate healing and brotherly love. In the mid-20th century, when green was proven to increase relaxation, hospitals redecorated with truckloads of pale green paint. Wearing green brings stability and balances your spiritual and material life. However, too much green solidifies rigid psychological patterns. Green's antiseptic properties destroy germs and prevent decay.

INCREASES	Healing, Balance, Stability, Harmony, Physical Relaxation, Calm, Serenity, Quietude, Soothing, Sedation, Expansiveness, Compassion, Compromise, Open-Heartedness, Unpossessiveness, Brotherly Love, Sympathy, Graciousness, Helpfulness, Uplifting Others, Comfort, Security, Prosperity
AGGRAVATES	Rigidity, Inflexibility, Fixed Patterns
HEALS	Heart Conditions, Sleep Disorders, Insomnia, Nervous System, Stagnation, Regret, Attachment, Tension, Anxiety, Mood Swings, Irritability, Exhaustion, Homesickness, Hypocrisy, Egotism, Covetousness, Lustfulness, Selfishness, Discouragement, Indecision, Brooding
STIMULATES	Liver, Gallbladder, Pituitary, Muscle Building, Tissue Building, Renewal, Rest, Repose, Recuperation, Rejuvenation, Inspiration, Motivation, Stability, Equilibrium, Security, Letting Go, Hope, Cleansing
SUITABLE FOR	Antiseptic Needs, Medical Uniforms, Medical Offices, Hospitals, Doctors' Attire, Nurses' Attire, Healing Rooms, Therapy Rooms, Counseling Rooms, Kitchen Decor, Bedroom Decor, Pajamas, Bed Sheets, Politics, World Affairs, Negotiation, Arbitration, Lawyers Offices, Courtrooms, Government Buildings

Blue Vibrations

A bright, clear blue sky evokes reverence and spiritual emotions. To the ancient Hebrews, blue represented revelation. It was the color of curtains in the Tabernacle,[5] the robe of the ephod, and coverings for holy objects in the Ark.[6] The heroic Biblical figure Mordecai wore blue and white royal garments.[7]

Blue is cooling and expansive. When walls were painted blue in one corporation, employees caught more colds and absenteeism increased. Amazingly, when the backs of secretaries' chairs were painted warm, bright orange, the cold feeling in the office suddenly reversed. Employees took off their jackets, and attendance rose to normal again.[8]

Whereas green relaxes your body, light blue tranquilizes your mind. In mental institutions, violent, aggressive patients placed in a blue chamber or treated with blue light quickly calmed down.[9] However, the blue-gray color of dismal rain clouds increases depression or "feeling blue."

INCREASES	Purification, Mental Relaxation, Spiritual Awareness, Calmness, Coolness, Quietude, Soothing, Restfulness, Tranquility, Patience, Peace, Content
AGGRAVATES	Cold, Muscle Cramps, Paralysis, Rheumatism, Hypertension, Arthritis, Tics, Tremors, Pain, Gauntness, Ungroundedness
HEALS	Jaundice, Infections, Burns, Cuts, Bruises, Stings, Itching, Hives, Fever, Inflammation, Hyperactivity, Overexcitement, Overstimulation, Irritation, Critical Mind, Anger, Annoyance, Disturbances, Worries, Anxieties
STIMULATES	Perspiration, Building Vitality, Antiseptics, Antibiotics, Reverence, Awe, Spirituality, Religious Emotion, Freedom, Creativity, Patience, Loyalty, Devotion, Harmony, Honesty
SUITABLE FOR	Antiseptic Needs, Bedroom Decor, Pajamas, Bed Sheets, Meditation Room, Meditation Attire, Church Decor, Clergy Attire, Spiritual Centers, Esoteric Bookstores, Medical Clothing, Doctors' Attire, Nurses' Attire, Janitors' Attire, Bathroom Decor, Laundromats, Creative Endeavors, Artists' Studios

Indigo and Purple Vibrations

Indigo or purple light evokes solemnity, a majestically inspired reverence in the presence of something deeply sublime and rare. Purple is traditionally the color of royalty. Indigo, a mystical color, augments spiritual experiences, develops intuition, and stimulates freedom, self-reliance, idealism, and divine direction. This is an idealistic color that helps you remember your true soul-purpose, goals, and dreams. Indigo can align your purpose to God's will. If you are too intellectual, indigo brings you into your intuitive nature. Indigo and purple are powerful sedatives to numb pain and overcome hyperactivity. However, too much indigo can magnify spaced-out feelings or restrict blood flow and raise blood pressure.

INCREASES	True Purpose, Heart's Desire, Realizing Goals, Realizing Ideals, Sedation, Anesthesia, Numbness to Pain, Intuition, Solemnity, Idealism
AGGRAVATES	Feeling Spaced-Out, Feeling Ungrounded, Blood Pressure
HEALS	Overexcitement, Hyperactivity, Fevers, Overactive Kidneys, Obsession, Fear, Repression, ADD
STIMULATES	Activity of Veins, Reverence, Awe, Spiritual Experience, Psychic Perception, Meditation, Self-Reliance, Free Expression, Self-Expression, Individualism
SUITABLE FOR	Church Decor, Palace Decor, Hotel Decor, Luxurious Decor, Clergy Attire, Royal Attire, Esoteric Centers, Esoteric Bookstores, Meditation Rooms, Meditation Attire, Psychics' Attire

Violet Vibrations

Violet enhances spiritual awareness, meditation, unconditional love for humanity, creative imagination, higher thoughts, ESP, and sensitivity to higher dimensions. The violet ray reverses petty anxieties and attachment to chains of materialism. Violet pacifies nerves and soothes high-strung people. In mental institutions, violet light or violet wall paint calmed or cured violent patients.[10] This color reduces the activity of organs and systems, such as heart, muscles, lymph, and nervous system.

Leonardo da Vinci said, "The power of meditation can be ten times greater under violet light falling through the stained-glass window of a quiet church." Renowned German composer Richard Wagner composed spiritual music behind violet curtains.[11]

INCREASES	Calm, Inspiration, Clarity, Spiritual Communication, Divine Realization, Divine Love, Humanitarianism, Brotherly Love, Psychic Perception, Telepathy, ESP, The Paranormal, Deeper Realities
AGGRAVATES	Feeling Spaced-Out, Feeling Ungrounded, Extremism
HEALS	Nerves, Blood, Scalp Diseases, Hunger, Oversensitivity, Overexcitement, Neurosis, Psychosis, Materialism
STIMULATES	Spleen Activity, Bone Growth, White Blood Cells, Blood Purification, Divine Creativity, Creative Imagination, Divine Contact, Higher Consciousness, Spiritual Emotions, Spiritual Awareness, Unconditional Love
SUITABLE FOR	Meditation Rooms, Creative Rooms, Artists' Studios, Music Studios, Symphony Halls, Churches, Religious Buildings, Esoteric Bookstores, Clergy Attire, Psychics' Attire, Psychics' Rooms, Appetite Suppression

White Vibrations

The pure white light of Spirit contains all the cosmic rays. Because white light is pure refected sunlight, it contains all colors. Blinding sunlight bathes everything in radiance, reveals and exposes everything, and dispels all shadows. Therefore white is unblemished—the purest color of absolute perfection. White light, which includes all colors in harmony, is the most mystical color. To the ancient Hebrews, white symbolized purity, innocence, and morality. Ancient priests wore white linen garments.

By imbibing white sunlight, your body is revitalized with all colors simultaneously. Moderate sunbathing absorbs pranic energies of all colors. As you lic in the sun, imagine pure white healing light rays energizing your organs and cells—especially where healing is needed. To increase spiritual energy, picture yourself surrounded with an aura of pure white luminous sphere of diamond-like brightness. At the same time, imagine you are in harmony with all life.

INCREASES	Spirituality, Mysticism, Perfection of Soul, Spiritual Qualities, Spiritual Awareness, Purity, Harmony, Innocence, Enlightenment, Creativity, Weight Loss
AGGRAVATES	Feeling Ungrounded, Dizziness, Perfectionism, Compulsion, Obsession, Mood Swings, Bipolar Disorder, Extremism, Fanaticism
HEALS	Disease, Toxins, Discomfort, Disharmony, Moral Decay, Impurity, Overstimulation, Disorder, Chaos, Stress, Vexation
STIMULATES	Detachment, Energy, Vitality, Healing, Morality, Ethics, Exposing Truth, Upliftment, Lofty Thoughts
SUITABLE FOR	Meditation Rooms, Churches, Clergy Attire, Tropical Climates, Keeping Cool, Summer Clothing, Cooling Ships, Cooling RVs, Cooling Vehicles, Cooling Buildings

Black Vibrations

Black, the absence of energy and light, absorbs all colors and reflects no light waves. Therefore black objects appear colorless, like a hole in light. To the ancient Hebrews, black symbolized death, humility, and mourning. Thus the bereaved wear black to mourn their loved ones. Whenever black is added to a color, the resulting shade symbolizes negative qualities. When you close your eyes, you see black as you shut out external stimuli. Therefore, black increases introversion and can be useful for withdrawing from overwhelming situations and for grounding. It can also enhance the practice of magic and in uncovering things hidden from view. When a round black rug is placed at an entryway, Alzheimer's patients will stay home and not wander. Teenagers who need grounding often like to wear black.

INCREASES	Silence, Inner Peace, Stopping Activity, Sadness, Grief, Mourning, Traditionalism, Conservatism
AGGRAVATES	Contraction, Isolation, Psychosis, Illness, Disease, Despair, Negativity, Despondency, Destructiveness, Defensiveness, Depression, Discouragement, Self-Indulgence, Sexual Deviance, Drug Abuse, Subculture Cultism, Escapism, Suicide, Astral Possession
HEALS	Overwhelm, Overstimulation, Intensity, Aggravation, Irritation
STIMULATES	Negatism, Energy Drain, Grief, Gloom, Magic Powers, Occult Knowledge, Nonconformity
SUITABLE FOR	Contrast, Background, Grounding, Deep Silence, Quietude, Rest, Rejuvenation, Containment, Shutting Others Out, Total Introversion, Uncovering Secrets, Clergy Attire, Formal Attire

Visualizing Color

Visualizing color is a powerful way to transform and lift your energy and heal your mind, body, and spirit. Your energy field is under your command, and you can control, regulate, or transform it through visualization.

Just before meditation or sleep, you can practice a form of mental chromotherapy. Close your eyes and make a mental picture of a sphere of color permeating and surrounding yourself, or another individual who needs healing. See that sheen of light as tangibly and powerfully as possible, in whatever color is suitable for the given situation. Then imagine the result you are attempting to achieve, such as radiant health, prosperity, joy, or otherwise. Then go into a deep state of meditation or fall asleep, bathed in that glow of color.

Just a little practice in visualizing color in your aura will demonstrate how powerfully your mind can change your mental, physical, and emotional state, regardless of your surroundings.

The Sounds of Colors

The seven colors of the spectrum are associated with letters of the alphabet, musical notes, planets, powers (*shaktis*), and power-sounds (*mantras*), as follows:[12]

Color	Red	Orange	Yellow	Green	Blue	Indigo	Violet
Musical Note	C, Do	D, Re	E, Mi	F, Fa	G, Sol	A, La	B, Ti
Letter	A	E	I	O	U	W	Y
Planet	Sun	Moon	Mars	Mercury	Jupiter	Venus	Saturn
Sanskrit Name	Surya	Chandra	Mangala	Budha	Guru	Shukra	Shani
Element	Fire	Water	Earth			Ether	Air
Shakti Power	Harana: Attracts	Sharana: Delights	Karana: Works	Vachana: Teaches	Starana: Expands	Kama: Loves	Stambhana: Delays, Stops
Mantra	Hreem	Shreem	Kreem	Aim	Streem	Kleem	Hleem

The correspondences of musical notes and colors were discovered through studies of clairvoyants who see particular colors when specific musical notes are played. For example, middle C is red, B is violet, and so forth. The note F-sharp is between green and blue, so it is turquoise. When chords are played, three colors manifest simultaneously. When notes are in higher octaves, colors become lighter. When lower octaves are played, colors are darker.

The qualities of each color match with their corresponding notes. For instance, the musical note C brings strength and vitality, the note G calms the mind, and so forth. So healing can occur when you hear particular notes or chords. Using sensitive instruments, scientists discovered that the sound of grass growing is the F note, corresponding to green. When the note F is played, grass grows healthier and faster.

Red, at the beginning of the spectrum, is associated with the sound in which your mouth opens to produce the most primal sound. The sound "Ah" is not only the first letter of the alphabet and first note of the musical scale. It is also the first sound of the Vedas of India, which are said to be the underlying vibrations that give rise to the universe.

The sound of orange, "Ee" is a metaphor for the quality of orange, which is a desire for fuller expression. This sound is produced when your tongue reaches up and out, seeking to combine with the palate.

The sound of yellow, the letter "I," represents your identity and individuality. It is the sound of the ego, the "I"—the full development of intellect that yellow represents.

The sound of the green vibration, "Oh," is associated with the exclamation of awe and wonder—the thrill resulting from inquiry or research, new experiences, traveling to new places, or seeing beauty. Green, the most soothing color, is associated with beauty.

The "U," or "You," sound, like the color blue, is the sound that reaches out to give rather than receive. Thus it is the sound of charity and moral, ethical, and spiritual values.

The sound "Wah" is made by pursing the lips into a tight circle. The low, somber, bass tone of this sound corresponds to the solemn, deep nature of indigo vibrations.

The "Y," or "Why," sound of violet is a metaphor for spiritual inquiry into higher reaches of human development. Violet vibrations indicate higher states of consciousness.

Mantras to Strengthen Your Energy Field

Traditionally in India, sounds called *mantras* are used to strengthen the energy field. A mantra is a vibrational sound that invokes a deity and produces particular known results.

Gayatri Mantra

Perhaps the most effective mantra for cleansing and healing your auric field is the *Savitri Gayatri* mantra, prayer to *Savitri,* the Solar Orb, found in *Rig-Veda,* III.62.10:

*Om Bhoor Bhuvah Swah Tat Savitu Varenyam Bhargo
Devasya Dheemahi Dhiyo Yo Nah Prachodayaat.*

Here is a translation of the Gayatri Mantra:

*"I meditate on the spiritual effulgence of that adorable light,
the ultimate reality, source of the universe and the three worlds
of physical, astral, and subtle planes—who is worthy of
praise. Unveil to me the face of the true spiritual sun, the
supreme Self, who appears through a disc of golden light.
May that divine being bless me, purify and illuminate my
intellect, guide my soul, and open my inner eye of wisdom,
that I may realize the ultimate truth."*

Chanting or meditating with this mantra at least 108 times each day invokes divine light to cleanse your energy field. This mantra has untold benefits, including acting in highest wisdom, speaking with sweetness, clarity of mind, greater discernment, following your true purpose, fulfilling your destiny, and attaining enlightenment.

When chanting mantras, people often use a rosary called a *mala* to count the number of repetitions, as it is generally recommended to chant mantras 108 times. Therefore you will find sandalwood, or *rudraksha* (a seed holy to Lord Shiva), malas with 108 beads. You can order rudraksha malas at *www.divinerevelation.org*.

Important Note: *Mispronouncing Sanskrit mantras can have deleterious results*. Before chanting any of the mantras in this chapter, if you are not knowledgeable about Sanskrit, please study with a teacher to clarify the pronunciation. Or order a CD of mantras at *www.divinerevelation.org*.

The following chart presents mantras that correspond with the planets, days of the week, gemstones, shapes, and colors governed by them. These mantras are invocations of the energies of the planets, and they are to be used on the weekday specified.

Weekday	Planet	Mantra	Color	Shape
Sunday	Sun	Aum hreem hansah sooryaaya namah	Red	Square, Rectangle
Monday	Moon	Aum kreem cham chandraye namah	Orange	Round
Tuesday	Mars	Aum baum bhaumaya namah	Yellow	Double-drum (Hourglass)
Wednesday	Mercury	Aum bum buddhaaya namah	Green	Triangle
Thursday	Jupiter	Aum braum brhaspataye namah	Blue	Ellipse
Friday	Venus	Aum kleem shum shukraya namah	Indigo	Octagon
Saturday	Saturn	Aum sham shanaishcharaaya namah	Violet	Square with Cross (4 Panes)
Saturday	Rahu North Node	Aum ram raahave namah	Black or Smoke	Stripes
Tuesday	Ketu South Node	Aum kem ketave namah	Brown or Smoke	Triangular Flag

Chant to the Supreme Light

Antar jyoti bahir jyoti pratyag jyoti parat parah
Jyotir jyoti swayam jyoti atma jyoti shivosmyaham.

Here is a translation of this mantra:

"Light is on the inside, light is on the outside, light is in myself, beyond the beyond. The Light of lights, I myself AM light, the Self is light, I AM Shiva!"

In the next chapter, you will learn profound breathing practices that powerfully increase your pranic energy in your auric field.

14

Using Breath With Intention

෨

Augmenting Pranic Energy

"To keep a light burning, we have to keep putting oil into it."
—Mother Teresa[1]

For thousands of years the yogis of India have recognized how increasing the life-force energy of prana can raise quality of life. Pranic energy is greatly enhanced through time-tested, ancient yogic practices of *pranayama* (breathing exercises).

In my books *Exploring Meditation* and *The Power of Chakras,* you will find many breathing exercises that are invaluable for augmenting prana and strengthening your aura. I urge you to refer to these books and learn these powerful secret yogic methods.

In this chapter I have included several esoteric breathing practices not mentioned in these previous books. Your aura can be healed, energized, and expanded through these profound methods, specifically designed to increase its power and brilliance.

Breath Is Life

From your first cry at infancy to your last gasp of death, your life is a long series of breaths. The yogis of India believe your lifespan is counted by the number of breaths, not the number of years. At birth you come into this world with a contract of a predetermined number of breaths. When these run out, your life is over. This is why conservation of breath is essential in yoga philosophy.

You may live for a long time without eating and for a short time without drinking water. But you will not live long if you don't breathe. By breathing consciously and deeply, you can boost vitality, strengthen resistance to disease, even extend your lifespan. By foolishly poisoning your pulmonary system through smoking, or by dissipating pranic energy through a profligate lifestyle, you will diminish vitality and shorten life.

Infants and children know how to breathe fully. They need no instruction. But this natural trait is lost in adults. Stooped shoulders, caved-in chests, and respiratory diseases (lung cancer, emphysema, and asthma) in epidemic proportions are the results of inadequate breathing practices.

A healthy routine of ample, complete breathing replete with prana, which nourishes every cell, can revitalize your life. Your energy field can be bright, powerful, and expanded. Your physical body can brim with vitality. You can become radiant and vigorous.

The yogis of India believe that proper breathing can annihilate all disease from this planet. In addition, the power of prana in breath can increase mental capacity, happiness, self-confidence, self-discipline, inner strength, and clarity, and can awaken latent mental powers. By controlling breathing through ancient secrets of pranayama, you can eliminate illness, let go of fear and worry, and unfold spiritual evolution.

How Breathing Revitalizes You

Your every breath is generated by a strong, sheet-like muscle separating your chest from your abdomen—your diaphragm. Its action creates a vacuum that forces air into your bronchial tubes, terminating in millions of minute air cells (*alveoli*) in your lungs which, if stretched out, would cover 14,000 square feet.

Life-giving oxygen penetrates the thin walls of the lungs' tiny blood vessels, where your blood absorbs oxygen and releases carbon dioxide from toxic waste matter gathered from your entire system. Every day, about 35,000 pints of blood pass through your lung capillaries in single file, corpuscle by corpuscle, while exposed to oxygen on both surfaces.

Once the blood is purified and oxygenated, bright red and infused with pranic energy, it travels to the left auricle of your heart. There it is forced into the left ventricle, where this rich, life-giving blood is pumped through your arteries and into your capillaries to nourish every part of your body.

Then bluish, dark red, dull blood, burdened with waste matter, returns through the capillaries into your veins and toward your heart and lungs, seeking replenishment. This polluted blood enters your heart's right auricle. When this chamber is filled, it forces blood into your heart's right ventricle and then into your lungs, where millions of tiny blood vessels distribute the blood into your lungs' miniscule air cells.

It is obvious that unless you get enough fresh air into your lungs, your blood will not be sufficiently purified or regenerated to maintain optimum health. It will assume a bluish-red color, and your complexion will acquire an unhealthy pallor. Blood impurities will manifest disease.

In fact, with oxygen starvation, the foul stream of venomous blood rushing through your veins cannot be purified. It poisons your system. Your body is robbed of nourishment, and death results.

In contrast, when your arterial blood contains about 25 percent oxygen, your body functions optimally. Every cell, tissue, muscle, and organ is invigorated and strengthened. New, pristine, healthy cells and tissues are easily manufactured.

Oxygenated blood, generated by deep breathing, increases body warmth, strengthens resistance, and brings proper food assimilation and waste elimination.

Yogic Pranayama

The air around you is charged with pranic energy, which is absorbed when you breathe. However, by controlling and regulating breathing, as yogis do, you can extract a far greater supply of prana. This powerful energy can be stored in your brain and energy centers (particularly your solar plexus), just as batteries store electricity.

Yogis know that by practicing secret breathing methods, called *pranaya-ma*, they can strengthen their body and also develop spiritual energy, psychic abilities, and latent powers. In fact, they can transfer this energy to heal and lift others.

The Sanskrit word *pranayama* derives from the roots *prana* ("moving" or "breathing forth") and *ayama* ("stretching," "extending," "restraining," or "expanding in time and space"). Thus, pranayama overcomes limitations, expands energy, and increases sensitivity to higher vibrations and dimensions. By eliminating mental distractions and internal conflicts, pranayama allows consciousness to shine in pristine purity, without distortion.

A fundamental principle of yogic pranayama is to inhale through your nostrils. Your nose, with its bristly hairs and warming mucous membrane, is the protective filter for your entire respiratory system. If you breathe in through your mouth, nothing sieves out the impurities, germs, foreign matter, and cold that is inhaled directly into your lungs.

Your energy field will attain greater vibrancy, expansion, strength, and energy when you practice the pranayama exercises in this chapter.

Yogic Complete Breathing

The yogis of India classify breathing into four basic categories: high breathing, middle breathing, low breathing, and yogic complete breathing. Let us now briefly explore these methods and learn how to practice each one.

High Breathing

High breathing, also known as clavicular or collarbone breathing, is commonly practiced by highly stressed, tense people. This method allows only a miniscule portion of air to enter the upper part of the chest and lungs. Your ribs, collarbone, and shoulders lift up, while your abdomen contracts and pushes up the diaphragm, preventing your lungs from expanding. High breathing uses maximum effort to achieve minimum results.

Try this experiment: Expel all the air from your lungs. Then stand erect with hands at your sides. Pull in your stomach muscles, and at that same time, raise your shoulders and collarbone as you inhale and exhale several times. You will discover the quantity of air that you inhale is grossly inadequate.

Middle Breathing

Also known as rib breathing or intercostal breathing, middle breathing allows more air to enter your nasal passages. Your diaphragm pushes upward and your abdomen draws inward. Your ribs rise up and your chest partially expands. Air fills only the middle part of your lungs, not your entire lungs. This inadequate breathing method is often taught by physical education trainers.

Try this experiment: Expel all the air from your lungs. Then stand erect with hands at your sides. Inhale while expanding your ribs, pulling in your abdomen, and lifting your diaphragm. More air will enter than through high breathing, yet your lungs will still not expand fully.

Low Breathing

Also known as abdominal breathing, deep breathing, or diaphragmatic breathing, low breathing fills the middle and lower parts of the lungs. The virtues of low breathing are extolled by voice trainers, acting teachers, and yoga teachers as the superior method of breathing. Yet low breathing does not allow air to fill every part of your lungs.

When practicing abdominal breathing, as you inhale, your ribs move outward and your diaphragm contracts and moves downward. This movement expands your lungs. Hence, the diaphragm is key to absorbing pranic energy during breathing.

Now try this experiment: Sit up straight. Take some deep breaths while moving your diaphragm downward (pushing out your stomach). Do not raise your chest or shoulders. Your belly will distend and become convex as you inhale. As you exhale, your belly will collapse and become concave.

Yogic Complete Breathing

High breathing fills your upper lungs. Middle breathing fills the middle and upper part of your lungs. Low breathing fills the lower and middle parts. Yogic complete breathing, however, fills every portion of your lungs. That is why it is the best method of respiration. It brings maximum benefit from minimum energy expenditure.

Complete breathing is fundamental to all the other breathing methods in this chapter. Before attempting any other pranayama practices, it is essential to master this method of breathing until it becomes second nature. This is the foundation upon which a powerful, healthy energy field is built.

Practicing complete breathing does not require filling the lungs to capacity with every single breath. You can master this practice by using complete breathing for just a few minutes several times a day, until it becomes your natural form of breathing.

How to Practice

Stand or sit erect. Breathe through your nostrils, inhaling steadily. First fill the lower part of your lungs by practicing lower breathing. Your diaphragm descends and contracts, and your abdomen distends. Then fill the middle part of your lungs by pushing out the lower ribs, breastbone, chest, and ribs in your front, sides, and back. Then fill the upper part of your lungs. Allow your upper chest to protrude and lift, including the uppermost pairs of ribs attached to your breastbone. In your final movement, your collarbone and shoulders lift slightly and your lower abdomen draws inward. This gives support to your lungs and fills the highest portion of your lungs with air.

After inhaling, retain your breath for a few seconds. Then exhale slowly, holding your chest in a firm, steady position as you contract your abdomen and lift it upward slowly. When the air is entirely exhaled, relax your chest and abdomen.

The three movements of lower, middle, and upper breathing are achieved in one continuous motion. Your entire chest cavity, starting from your diaphragm and ending at your collarbone, moves as one uniform, undulating wave. Avoid jerky inhalations and strive for a steady, smooth, continuous motion. With some practice, the movement will become automatic.

Practice the complete breath before a large mirror. Place your hands lightly over your abdomen in order to feel its movements.

Important: As you practice this full yogic breath, never strain; take it easy. In the beginning, do not try to advance too quickly by inhaling forcefully or by practicing excessively.

Yogic Cleansing Breath

The key to full yogic breathing is to empty the lungs fully on the exhale so maximum prana can enter the lungs on the inhale. This secret method of Yogic Cleansing Breath ventilates and cleanses the lungs and refreshes the entire energy field. Often yogis use this breathing exercise at the end of pranayama practice. In this book you will use this method repeatedly. So practice and learn it now.

How to Practice

Inhale a complete breath. Retain the air for a few seconds. Then pucker your lips as though you are preparing to whistle. This is called "crow's beak gesture." Then blow out a little air with great vigor. Stop for a moment and retain the air. Then blow out a little more air with force. Repeat this process until all the air is exhaled from your lungs.

Yogic Retained Breath

Occasional breath retention is beneficial to the respiratory, digestive, and circulatory systems. Retaining breath absorbs waste matter, and expelling the air cleanses your lungs.

How to Practice

Stand erect and inhale a complete breath. Retain the air as long as you can comfortably hold it. Exhale vigorously through your open mouth. Then practice the Yogic Cleansing Breath as described on pages 226–227.

Yogic Sniff-Breathing

This yogic breathing method is a refreshing stimulant when you only have a few moments. It strengthens your lungs, brings relaxation and energy, and combats fatigue and emotional disturbances. It rejuvenates your spirit and improves coordination.

How to Practice

Stand erect or sit erect with spine in alignment. Exhale fully. Then, as you breathe in, instead of inhaling in one steady stream, take a series of short, quick sniffs. Continue to retain your breath and do not exhale as you continue to add sniffs of air until your lung space is completely filled. Then retain your breath for a few seconds. Breathe out through your mouth with a long, restful sigh. Then practice the Yogic Cleansing Breath on page 226.

Yogic Rhythmic Breathing

Rhythmic breathing attunes you to life's vibrations and harmonizes your body with nature's rhythms. In this way you can absorb, store, and control vast resources of prana.

Rhythmic breathing is based on pulse beats. By placing your fingers on your wrist or neck, you can feel your pulse. For the beginner, inhale for a count of six pulse beats. You can gradually increase this number through regular practice.

How to Practice

In this method, the number of beats for inhalation and exhalation are equal. After inhaling, you will retain your breath for half of that number, as follows:

Sit erect in an easy posture. Hold your chest, neck, and head in a straight line. Inhale slowly a complete breath as you count six pulse beats. Retain your breath for three pulse beats. Then exhale slowly through your nostrils for six pulse beats. Count three pulse beats before you take your next breath. Repeat this several times, without straining. After you complete this exercise, practice the Yogi Cleansing Breath on page 226.

After a few months of practice, gradually increase the duration of inhalations and exhalations to 16 pulse beats with eight pulse beats for retention.

Important: Do not strain and try to increase the breath interval too quickly. Harmonious rhythm is more important than duration. Slow and steady is the rule for developing your capacity for pranayama. Otherwise you might damage delicate lung tissues.

Yogic Rhythmic Breathing With Mental Focus

Once you become proficient at Yogic Rhythmic Breathing, your interval of inhale and exhale becomes automatically regulated without counting pulse beats. Then you can add mental focus or visualization. Here are a few pranic exercises that use your creative imagination:

Distributing Prana

This exercise increases energy in your aura, especially when you feel tired or drained. Lie on your back on an exercise mat or on a bed, completely relaxed. Lightly rest your hands over your solar plexus, just above your navel. Practice rhythmic breathing. After your rhythm becomes regulated, then imagine that on every inhale, you are drawing an increased supply of prana or vital energy from the universal supply. See this inrushing pranic energy absorbed by your lungs, distributed by your nervous system, and stored in your solar plexus.

With every exhale, visualize your pranic energy distributed all over your body, to every organ, muscle, cell, atom, nerve, artery, and vein, from the top of your head to your fingertips, soles of feet, and toes. See this pranic energy invigorating and stimulating every pranic center, sending energy and strength throughout your system. Simply create a mental picture, without straining.

Healing Yourself of Illness

Lie down in a relaxed position and breathe rhythmically. Imagine enormous pranic energy being inhaled. With some exhalations, visualize sending pranic energy to the ailing area to stimulate and heal it. With alternate exhalations, imagine the diseased condition being expelled from your body.

Place both hands over the ill portion of your body. See pranic energy flowing down your arms, through your fingertips and palms, into your body. Without straining, gently hold the mental image that as you exhale, prana is pumped into your body through your hands. Imagine this energy stimulating your cells, driving out disease.

Healing Others of Illness

Sit erect. Breathe rhythmically while you imagine absorbing vast amounts of pranic energy for the purpose of transmitting that energy to a person in need of healing. Continue rhythmic breathing as you gently place your hands on or near the ailing portion of that individual's body. Stroke the body gently with fingertips or palms, or hold your hands near the body without touching it—however you feel led.

Form a clear mental image of a great influx of pranic energy pouring into your being. This energy flows down your arms, out your palms and fingertips, and into the body of the individual. As you breathe rhythmically, feel pranic energy pouring into the ill person's body in a continual, inexhaustible stream. Imagine that you are the pumping machinery connecting the person with the unending, universal supply of prana. See the body filled with pranic energy, stimulating weak organs and cells, imparting health, driving out disease, and stimulating cells. Allow this energy to flow through you freely as you continue rhythmic breathing.

You may choose to speak some affirmations aloud or silently, such as:

- ♨ "You are filled with pranic energy."
- ♨ "Prana is healing and lifting this seeming disease."
- ♨ "Prana is pervading and saturating your body now."
- ♨ "You are healed, strengthened, and invigorated by the power of prana now."
- ♨ "Your body is filled with life energy, light, healing, and pranic power now."

Occasionally raise your hands and flick your fingers, as though you were expelling disease from your hands. When the treatment is complete, wash your hands to avoid absorbing residual traces of the disease. Then practice the Yogic Cleansing Breath several times.

Feel free to vary these instructions to suit any particular client's needs.

Distant Healing

Using pranic energy, you can project healing at a distance to anyone who requests it. Your projected thought can be received through the ethers. To practice this, sit erect, yet relaxed. Create a mental picture of the person or call forth his/her essence and establish rapport—a sense of nearness to him/her. Once rapport is established, you can say mentally, *I send you a supply of vital force or power to invigorate and heal you.*

Now begin rhythmic breathing. With each exhale, imagine an infinite source of prana leaving your mind, traveling across space instantaneously, and reaching and healing the person in need. Imagine prana pumping into the person in an endless, continual stream. Imagine connecting the person to the universal, incessant supply of pranic energy. Allow this energy to flow through you freely as you continue rhythmic breathing. You may choose to speak some affirmations aloud or silently, as in the previous section on healing others.

Creating Pranic Thought-Forms

Projecting a Protective Shield

If you find yourself in situations where people are draining, manipulating, or harming you, or if you sense low vibratory energies or the influence of people's thoughts, then practice rhythmic breathing several times. Imagine you are generating a limitless power supply of pranic energy from the infinite source. Then see yourself surrounded with an egg-shape pranic aura, protecting you from gross thought-forms and disturbing vibrations.

Recharging Your Energy

If you feel low vitality or energy drain and you need a fresh supply quickly, then cross one ankle over the other. Interlace the fingers of your two hands together. This closes a pranic circuit and keeps vital energy from escaping through your extremities. While in this position, breathe rhythmically a few times to recharge your energy.

Charging Water and Food With Prana

Breathe rhythmically while holding a glass of water in your left hand. Imagine absorbing pranic energy and concentrating that energy into the fingertips of your right hand. Gently shake the fingertips of your right hand over the water, while visualizing pranic energy dropping into the water from your fingertips. After charging the water with prana this way, drink it or give it to someone needing healing. While drinking it, imagine the water is filled with pranic energy. The same system can be used to charge food before eating it.

Pranic Sexercise

The sexual energy that creates human life is a powerful vital force. This highly concentrated pranic energy can either generate new life or it can regenerate your own life. Enormous condensed pranic energy is amassed in your reproductive organs—the most powerful storage batteries in your physical body. The colossal force of sexual energy can be preserved to heal, strengthen, and vitalize your system. Or it can be expended in sexual activities and reproduction.

People with strong sexual energy have brilliant, large, healthy auras. When sexual energy is weak or dissipated, the aura becomes small, constricted, and murky. Sexual energy can increase prana in your subtle body and bring luster to your physical body.

The lore of ancient India speaks of the elixir of immortality, called *soma*, which originates from *ojas*, a sweet-smelling blood-product of a body and mind in a state of purity. Upon spending a long time in deep, silent meditation, try rubbing your face just as you come out. A somewhat greasy substance, called ojas, with a sweet-smelling fragrance, may cover your palms.

Ojas results in an auric emanation of brilliance, radiance, effulgence, and charisma. Ojas is a product of genital fluids, which are products of the marrow, which is a product of blood, which is, in turn, the product of food and oxygen.

By conserving genital fluids and transmuting sexual energy, you can nourish your endocrine glands with internal genital secretions. Those who practice secret methods of sexual energy conservation are filled with tremendous vital force and radiate powerful personal magnetism.

Since time immemorial yogis have known that sexual energy is a powerful tool that can benefit or harm. It is well-known that the spiritual life force energy in your body can flow upward to awaken and elevate your consciousness, or downward to satisfy sexual urges.

Instead of dissipating this treasure-trove of energy, you can revitalize and strengthen your system with it. Here is a breathing exercise that uses this powerful force to lift your vibration, amplify your energy field, and increase vital energy. Practice this anytime, especially when you are feeling sexual urges.

How to Practice

On pages 228 to 229 you learned how to practice rhythmic breathing. Lie passively or sit with your spine in a straight line. Practice rhythmic breathing and fix your mind on pranic energy, rather than sexual thoughts or fantasies. If these thoughts appear, do not be concerned. Simply realize this powerful energy can be used to strengthen your body and mind.

Visualize drawing this powerful subtle pranic energy from your genitals up into your solar plexus, where it will be transmuted and stored as a powerful reserve of vital force. Draw up this energy into the solar plexus with each inhale. You will feel pranic energy increasing in your solar plexus area.

You can also imagine the energy going to your heart for greater love and compassion, or to your brain for more intelligence, concentration, and supernormal powers. Use this energy for creative endeavors by imagining prana being drawn up with each inhale and sent forth in creative expression with each exhale.

Yogic Grand Spiritual Breath

This breathing exercise fills your entire system with prana most powerfully. It requires the lung capacity and mental capacity developed by practicing the previous exercises for several months. Therefore, first master the other exercises before attempting this one. When this is practiced with intention, you will feel as though you had a new body, freshly created, from head to toe.

How to Practice

Lie down in a relaxed, comfortable position. Practice rhythmic breathing until you have established a perfect rhythm. Visualize your pranic energy increasing. Picture this pranic energy breathing through the bones of your legs. Your breath is drawn upon through your bones with each inhale and then forced out of them with each exhale. Then imagine this energy in the same way through the bones of your arms. Then through the top of your skull. Through your stomach. Through your reproductive region. Imagine it traveling up and down along your spinal column. Visualize it inhaled and exhaled through every pore of your skin. Your whole body is filling with prana and life.

Then, as you continue to breathe rhythmically, send currents of prana to your vital centers. Use the internal mental image as before: Through the top of your head. Through your forehead. Through the back of your head. Through the base of your skull. Through the region of your neck. Through your heart area. Through your navel. Through your reproductive region. Through the base of your spine. Finish this exercise by sweeping the current of prana from head to foot several times.

Then practice the Yogic Cleansing Breath.

In the next chapter, you will augment your energy field through simple energetic movements that anyone can practice.

15

Using Energetic Movement

ကို

Vitalizing Your Energy Body

"Only the light which we have kindled in ourselves can illuminate others."

—Arthur Schopenhauer[1]

Today many people are overweight or plagued with various ailments, including hypertension, exhaustion, allergies, asthma, a compromised immune system, and chronic fatigue syndrome. Much of this suffering is caused by a sedentary lifestyle and a diet of highly processed foods. This difficulty is not just physical, however; it is also energetic. That is why working with the energy field and subtle body is so vital.

We can draw upon ancient wisdom to find solutions to our modern dilemma. By practicing simple movements, our energy field can be augmented, healed, lifted, and cleansed. Health can be restored quickly through concentrated effort. Please refer to my books *Exploring Meditation* and *The Power of Chakras* to learn yoga postures (*asanas*), yogic energy locks (*bandhas*), "Couch Potato Yoga," and other powerful energy practices.

In this chapter you will learn some additional exercises that produce powerful, immediate, beneficial results for transforming your energy field. All of these practices are simple to learn and practice. I guarantee that if you practice these simple movements daily, your life will improve.

Energy Warm-Up

The following 12-step, three-minute, simple Energy Warm-Up delivers immediate positive results. This exercise stimulates pranic flow throughout your system and increases energy in your field. Practice these simple tapping or rubbing movements to help you think more clearly and to increase inner strength, confidence, and positivism. They also protect you from negative emotions, thought-forms, and other atmospheric energies. In just three minutes, transform your mind, body, and spirit. Practice it now.

Important Note: Right before practicing these exercises, it is essential to drink enough fresh water until you feel fully hydrated.

1. Using two or three fingertips of one hand, tap or rub the cushiony area on the outside of your hand, for about 10 seconds. This point is halfway between where the little finger begins and the wrist bends. Switch hands and tap or rub your other hand. This relieves stress and calms your body.

2. Tap or rub the sides of each finger near the end of the nail bed for about 10 seconds. This balances your internal organs.

3. Tap or rub the back of your hand between the ring and pinky finger near your knuckle for about 10 seconds. At the same time, alternately look up and down, left and right, and diagonally, from side to side. This balances your brain. As you do this, hum to access your right brain, and then count from one to 10 to access your left brain.

4. Using three fingertips of both hands, tap or rub the top of your head in the area of your soft spot, the place where your parietal bones come together, for about 10 seconds.

5. Using two or three fingertips of both hands, tap or rub just above the beginning or wide section of your eyebrows, above left eyebrow with left fingers and above right eyebrow with right fingers, for about 10 seconds.

6. Using two or three fingertips of both hands, firstly on the bone bordering the outer corner of the eyes, and secondly about one inch under each eye, tap or rub for about 10 seconds in each spot.

7. Tap or rub under your nose (above your upper lip) and under your lower lip, for about 10 seconds. This stimulates the central and governing meridians of your body.

8. Using three fingertips of both hands, tap or rub the section of your collarbone closest to your breastbone, the left collarbone with the left fingers, and the right collarbone with the right fingers, for about 10 seconds.

9. Make a fist and tap or rub your breastbone in the center of your chest, for about 10 seconds. This stimulates your thymus gland, brings greater pranic energy to your body, and increases your strength and stamina.

10. With both hands, tap or rub the sides of your body just below your armpits for about 10 seconds.

11. Begin at the back of your head and stroke down your spine. This is a spinal flush, which will energize you. It will also remove toxins, waste, and stagnant energies from your system.

12. "Zip up" your energy body by drawing an imaginary zipper from your pubic bone all the way up to your chin. Do this three times in a row; the third time, make a motion as though you were turning a key to lock it.

Neck Activation

Stand up straight with feet together and hands at your sides. Open your eyes and relax your neck. Jerk your head, rotating toward your right shoulder as far as you can, and look toward the right as far as possible. Then jerk your head, rotating toward your left shoulder, and look left. Repeat at least 10 times.

Next, jerk your head forward to touch the sternal notch and backward to the nape of the neck. Repeat at least 10 times.

Then, keeping your chin in, try to touch your right shoulder with your right ear. Then try to touch left shoulder with left ear. While doing this, do not raise your shoulders. Repeat at least 10 times.

Lastly, keeping your chin in, rotate your head in circles, clockwise and counterclockwise, at least five times.

Shoulder Activation

Place arms at your sides with palms facing inward, toward your thighs. Tuck your thumbs into clenched fists. Pout your mouth into a small circle as though you are about to whistle. Suck in air and blow out your cheeks. Hold your breath and lower your chin to the sternal notch. Keeping your back straight and arms stiff as boards, pump your shoulders vigorously up and down as many times as possible while holding your breath. Do not bend your elbows. Then raise your head, open your eyes, relax your arms, and exhale slowly through your nose.

Brain Gym Exercises

Brain Gym is a series of easy movements developed by Paul E. Dennison, PhD, and Gail E. Dennison. As creators of Edu-Kinesthetics and pioneers in applied brain research, they created a system that I have found to be extremely powerful, yet exceedingly simple.

The five Brain Gym movements included here are from their book *Brain Gym Teacher's Edition*. The Dennisons explain that from infancy through adulthood, all brain activation occurs through movement. They further note that the simple, playful, and practical Brain Gym activities are a small part of the Educational Kinesiology learning-through-movement program, used in homes, schools, sports facilities, and businesses in more than 80 countries, and that these processes are especially useful for honoring the learner's natural pace and enhancing academic performance.

For more information about the Brain Gym curriculum, or for the name of a qualified instructor, please contact Brain Gym International at *www.braingym.org*. Brain Gym is a registered trademark of the Educational Kinesiology Foundation.

Important Note: Right before practicing these exercises, it is essential to drink enough fresh water until you feel fully hydrated.

Brain Buttons[2]

The Brain Buttons (soft tissue under the clavicle to the left and right of the sternum) are massaged deeply with one hand while holding the navel with the other hand.

Teaching Tips

- The student stimulates these points for 20 to 30 seconds, or until any tenderness is released.

- The Brain Buttons may be tender at first; over a few days to a week, the tenderness subsides. Even then, holding the points will activate them.

- The student may change hands to activate both brain hemispheres.

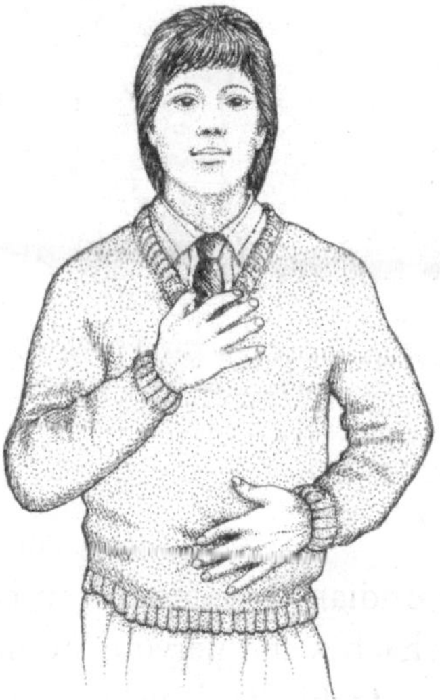

History of the Movement

Brain Buttons lie directly over and stimulate the carotid arteries that supply freshly oxygenated blood to the brain. The brain,

Figure 15a.[3]

though one-fiftieth of the body weight, uses one-fifth of its oxygen. Placing a hand on the navel re-establishes the gravitational center of the body, balancing the stimulus to and from the semicircular canals (centers of equilibrium in the inner ear). Dyslexia and related learning difficulties are associated with misinterpreted directional messages, known in Applied Kinesiology to be caused in part by visual inhibition. Brain Buttons establish a kinesthetic base for visual skills, whereby the ability to cross the body's lateral midline is dramatically improved.

The Positive Points[4]

The student lightly touches the point above each eye with the fingertips of each hand. The points are on the frontal eminences, as illustrated in the following figure, just above the eyeballs, halfway between the hairline and the eyebrows.

Teaching Tips

- The student thinks of something he would like to remember, such as the spelling of a word, or concentrates on a potentially stress-producing situation, such as a spelling test.

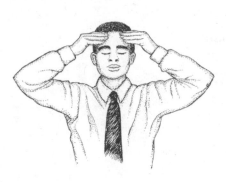

Figure 15b.[5]

๑ The student closes his eyes and allows himself to experience the image or experience the associated tension and then its release.

History of the Movement

The Dennisons renamed these emotional stress-release points from Touch for Health the Positive Points. These points are the neurovascular balance points for the stomach meridian. People tend to hold stress in the abdomen, resulting in stomachaches and nervous stomachs, a pattern often established in early childhood while sophisticated cortical development is taking place. The Positive Points bring blood flow from the hypothalamus to the frontal lobes, where rational thought occurs. This prevents the fight-or-flight response, so that a new response to the situation can be learned.

Lazy 8s[6]

Drawing the Lazy 8 or infinity symbol enables the reader to cross the visual midline without interruption, thus activating both right and left eyes and integrating the right and left visual fields. The 8 is drawn on its side and includes a definite midpoint and separate left and right areas, joined by a continuous line.

Teaching Tips

๑   The student aligns her body with a point at eye level. This will be the midpoint of the 8.

๑   The student chooses a comfortable position for drawing the Lazy 8, adjusting the width and height to fit her needs. (It is best to involve one's full visual field and the full extension of both arms.)

๑   The student may use the left hand first, to activate the right hemisphere immediately.

    ⚀ She starts on the midline and moves counterclockwise first: up, over, and around. Then, from her waist, she moves clockwise: up, over, around, and back to the beginning midpoint.

    ⚀ As the eyes follow the Lazy 8, the head moves slightly and the neck remains relaxed.

    ⚀ Three repetitions with each hand separately, then with both together, are recommended. Two colors of chalk or ink may be used.

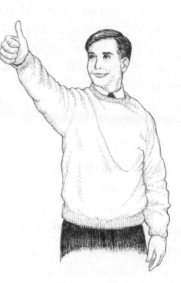

Figure 15c.[7]

Variations

    ⚀ The student may do the movement with eyes closed to increase her kinesthetic sense of the Lazy 8.

    ⚀ Humming while doing the Lazy 8 may increase relaxation.

    ⚀ Draw the Lazy 8 in the air with streamers, or against different tactile surfaces such as sand, paper, or chalkboard.

    ⚀ Graduate the 8 from larger to smaller sizes, drawn first on a large surface parallel to the face, and later, at a desk, so the movement is connected to writing.

    ⚀ Energy 8's: Swing both arms simultaneously down, across each other, then up and over. Move arms slowly, being aware of both left and right visual fields, and then quickly, soft-focusing on the afterimage of the arms.

History of the Movement

Tracing or feeling movement along a small infinity symbol, or Lazy 8, has been used in educational therapy to develop kinesthetic and tactile awareness in students with severe learning problems. These students are not yet ready neurologically to cross the visual midline. The movement results in the elimination of reversals and transpositions in reading and writing. Dr. Dennison adapted the Lazy 8 as part of his vision-training work in 1974 by having students use their large muscles to draw Lazy 8s on the chalkboard, the eyes following the hand movements. His students showed immediate improvement in the ability to discriminate symbols and to know their left from their right sides.

The Cross Crawl[8]

In this contralateral exercise, similar to walking in place, the student alternately moves one arm and its opposite leg and the other arm and its opposite leg. Because Cross Crawl accesses both brain hemispheres simultaneously, this is the ideal warm-up for all skills that require crossing the body's lateral midline.

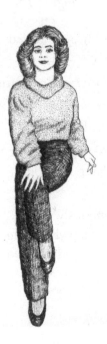

Figure 15d.[9]

Teaching Tips

♪   Water and Brain Buttons help prepare the body and brain to respond to Cross Crawl.

♪   To activate the kinesthetic sense, alternately touch each hand to the opposite knee.

Variations

♪   Cross Crawl as you sit, moving the opposite arm and leg together.

♪   Reach behind the body to touch the opposite foot.

♪   Do a slow-motion Cross Crawl, reaching opposite arm and leg to their full extension (Cross Crawl for focus).

& Skip or bounce lightly between each Cross Crawl. (Skip-Across is especially helpful for centering; it also alleviates visual stress.)

& To improve balance, Cross Crawl with your eyes closed, or pretend to swim while Cross Crawling.

& Do Cross Crawl to a variety of music and rhythms.

History of the Movement

As the body grows, interweaving of the opposite sides through movement naturally occurs during such activities as crawling, walking, and running. Over the last century, crawling has been used in neurological patterning to maximize learning potential. Experts theorized that contralateral movements worked by activating the speech and language centers of the brain. However, Dr. Dennison discovered that Cross Crawl activity is effective because it stimulates the receptive as well as expressive hemisphere of the brain, facilitating integrated learning. This preference for whole-brain movement over one-side-at-a-time processing can be established through Dennison Laterality Repatterning (see *Edu-K for Kids*).

Hook-Ups[10]

Hook-ups connect the electrical circuits in the body, containing and thus focusing both attention and disorganized energy. The mind and body relax as energy circulates through areas blocked by tension. The figure 8 pattern of the arms and legs (Part One) follows the energy flow lines of the body. The touching of the fingertips (Part Two) balances and connects the two brain hemispheres.

Teaching Tips

& Part One: Sitting, the student crosses the left ankle over the right. He extends his arms before him, crossing the left wrist over the right. He then interlaces his fingers and draws his hands up toward his chest. He may now close his eyes, breathe deeply, and relax for about a minute. Optional: He presses his tongue flat against the roof of his mouth on inhalation, and relaxes the tongue on exhalation.

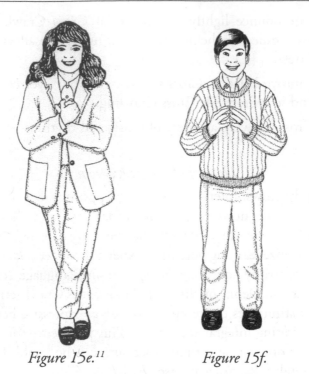

Figure 15e.[11]   *Figure 15f.*

⚘ Part Two: When ready, the student uncrosses his legs. He touches the fingertips of both hands together, continuing to breathe deeply for about another minute.

Variations

⚘ Hook-ups may also be done while sitting or standing.

⚘ For Part One, some people may prefer to place the right ankle and right wrist on top.

History of the Movement

Hook-ups shift electrical energy from the survival centers in the hindbrain to the reasoning centers in the midbrain and neocortex, thus activating hemispheric integration, increasing fine-motor coordination, and enhancing formal reasoning. Developmentally, such integration pathways are usually established in infancy through sucking and cross-motor movement. The tongue pressing into the roof of the mouth stimulates the limbic system for emotional processing in concert with more refined reasoning in the frontal lobes.

Excessive energy to the receptive (right or hind) brain can manifest as depression, pain, fatigue, or hyperactivity. This energy gets redirected in Part One to the expressive (left) brain in a figure-8 pattern. Dr. Dennison discovered that this posture could also be used to release emotional stress and alleviate learning difficulties. Wayne Cook, an expert in electromagnetic energy, invented a variation of this posture, from which Hook-ups are adapted, as a way to counterbalance the negative effects of electrical pollution.

The books *Brain Gym Teacher's Edition* and *Brain Gym for Business*, where you can learn dozens of Brain Gym exercises and get detailed information about each exercise, are available at *www.divinerevelation.org*.

In the next chapter, you will learn how to use dowsing tools to increase energy in your aura and your surroundings and to heal detrimental energies.

16

Using Intuitive Kinesiology

ಬಿ

Tools to Strengthen Your Aura

"Within you is the light of the world. It must be shared with the world."

—Peace Pilgrim[1]

In Arosa, Switzerland, in 1974, I was serving on the personal staff of my guru, Maharishi Mahesh Yogi. The first time I ever saw a pendulum was the day Daniel Maurin, a French healer, visited our ashram. Daniel invited me to sit next to him, and he swung his pendulum, a squashed slice of bread at the end of string, over a multi-colored pie chart. (Yes, you read that right: bread on a string!) He made notations and then handed me several curious glass tubular vials. To open them, I had to break their ends. One was labeled Uranium.

The bizarre, mysterious remedies lasted about a month. To my great surprise, I never felt so healthy, robust, positive, and powerful as during that single month in 1974. Brimming with energy, I barely slept. I certainly wish I could find a healer like Daniel Maurin again.

Your Imagination: Your Only Limitation

In 1982, a county office building in Butte, California, was built with no vent ducts in the air-conditioning system. No fresh air circulated through the building, and the windows did not open. In the assessor's office of 50 employees, the sick rate increased by 1.5 percent. Houseplants drooped.

Tony Gehringer, a master dowser from Las Cruces, New Mexico, was the assessor's assistant at the time. With his pendulum, he used a pie chart similar to the ones provided in this chapter to measure air quality in the building, which tested negative 8 on a scale from negative 10 to positive 10. Oxygen content was 8 percent but should have been 20 percent.

Tony and Walt Woods, another master dowser, decided that their only limitation was their imagination, or lack thereof. So, with a pendulum, they asked whether their higher self could permanently transform the air quality in the building to resemble a forest near a stream of water. They were amazed to receive a Yes response. As they continued to work with a pendulum daily, eventually the air quality substantially improved until it measured positive 10 and oxygen content measured 20 percent.

During the next quarter, the sick rate decreased. By the end of the following quarter, the sick rate returned to normal. Houseplants became robust. Employees no longer fell ill. The building's air quality remained excellent until Tony retired in 1984.

Because your only limitation is your imagination, let us now see what miraculous results you can create using your own Intuitive Kinesiology tools.

Pendulum Auric Healing

When you use a pendulum, the sky is the limit. Many skillful pendulumists create stunning results in all areas of life. Some serve clientele all over the world, locating potable water or finding lost objects through map dowsing. They perform incredible healings with charts similar to those in this chapter.

Important Note: Before attempting any of the processes below, first read and study Chapter 6. Complete the Warm-Up Exercises on page 236 right before each process.

Pendulum Percentage Chart

Let us do our first experiment now. Refer to Figure 16a (Pendulum Percentage Chart). Place this chart on a table. After completing the Warm-Up Exercises, place your pendulum in the Ready position. In this chart, Ready position is swinging to the left. Then say to your higher self audibly,

Pendulum Percentage Chart

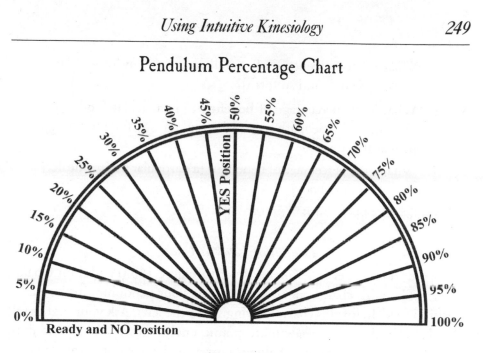

Figure 16a.

"Please indicate my current percentage of optimum aura health and balance." Take a deep breath and let go. Your pendulum will then move through the chart until it consistently swings in one of the pie-sections, indicating your current percentage of optimum aura health and balance.

Once you determine this figure, swing your pendulum in the Ready position again. Ask your higher self audibly, "Can my higher self make beneficial corrections at this time?" If you get a No answer (continuing to swing to the left), then do not proceed. If you get a Yes answer (swinging forward and backward), then tell your higher self aloud, "Please bring my aura into optimum health and balance."

Then swing your pendulum in the Ready position over the chart. The pendulum will move from the Ready position, through the chart, while your aura achieves the maximum optimum health and balance possible at this time. If it is not 100 percent, then continue to work with your pendulum daily until your aura attains 100-percent optimum health and balance.

Now is time to exercise your imagination. What other measurements and corrections can you make with this chart? Remember: You can ask your higher self anything—even to improve the nutritious value of the food on your plate.

Here are just a few sample questions:

1. What is the percentage of overall health of my [dog, plant, sister, husband, and so forth]?

2. What is the percentage of benefit of [a particular food, vitamin, herb, homeopathic remedy, and so on] for my energy field at this time?

3. What is the percentage of benefit of [a particular holistic healer] to work on my body?

You get the idea, right?

Pendulum Chakra Chart

Let us do another experiment. Refer to Figure 16b (Pendulum Chakra Chart). Place this chart on a table and swing your pendulum in the Ready position (which, for this chart, is swinging to the left). Ask your higher self aloud: "Which chakra needs more pranic energy now?" Your pendulum will move to indicate which chakra is currently depleted of pranic energy.

Then move to Figure 16a and ask your higher self, "What is the current percentage of pranic energy in the [name of chakra needing energy]?" Your pendulum will move to indicate the current percentage.

Pendulum Chakra Chart

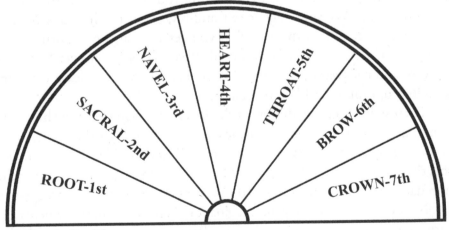

Ready Position

Figure 16b.

Swing your pendulum in the Ready position and then ask your higher self, "Can you make beneficial corrections in my [name of chakra needing energy] chakra now?" If you get a "yes" response, return to Ready position and tell your higher self, "Please make the beneficial corrections and bring optimum pranic energy into this [name of chakra needing energy] now." Your pendulum will move to make corrections and then indicate the percentage of energy now infused into that particular chakra.

Now turn back to Figure 16b and ask your higher self again whether another chakra needs pranic energy. Repeat the previous instructions until you have infused pranic energy into whatever chakras need energy.

Pendulum Color Chart

The Pendulum Color Chart (Figure 16c) can determine your current aura color or any other possible information about color. Use the color chart to ask any of the following questions, or any other questions you can conceive of:

1. What is the primary color of my aura now?

2. What color is depleted in my auric field that would be beneficial for me to increase now?

Pendulum Color Chart

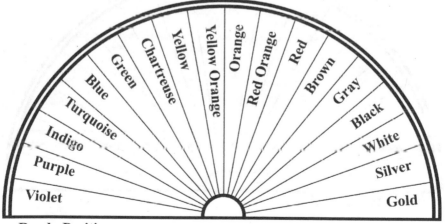

Figure 16c.

3. What color would be beneficial for me to wear today?

4. What color light would be beneficial to project onto my [root chakra area, sacral chakra area, and so on]?

5. What color would be beneficial for healing this [flu, cold, allergy, impotence, overweight, hypertension, and so forth]?

After determining what color is needed in your energy field, turn to Figure 16a to measure its current percentage in your field. Then ask your higher self to make beneficial adjustments. Also, refer to Chapter 13 for information about using colored light, color-infused water, and so forth.

Pendulum Write-In Chart

Use Figure 16d to determine anything else you want to test or measure. Make photocopies of this chart and write in whatever you want to ask about. Remember: your only limitation is your imagination.

Note: Dowsing tools are not diagnostic or curative tools. Consult a qualified medical professional for guidance and supervision to test or measure physical health and before using any healing modality.

Pendulum Write-In Chart

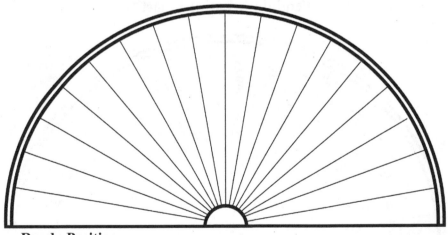

Ready Position

Figure 16d.

How to Heal and Balance an Aura

Here is a simple way to measure, balance, and heal the energy field of another person using one L-rod. (Note: this will not work with two L-rods.)

After doing the Warm-Up Exercises, ask someone to stand about 5 feet away from you. Place one L-rod in Ready position and tell your higher self, "Please show me the outer surface of this person's mental body." Move slowly toward the person until your L-rod moves into Found position to indicate the outer edge of the mental/emotional body.

Then measure around the front, back, left, right, head, and foot of your subject. Keep your L-rod steady, pointing slightly downward at about a 5-degree angle. You might find the shape of the aura is lopsided and/or unequal around the body. This indicates negative energies, influences, entities, or physical problems.

Then ask the person to lift his/her arms sideways while you slowly, systematically scan the entire energy field with your L-rod, searching for holes or depressions. Scan the head separately from the body. When you come to a hole, the L-rod will abruptly point inward toward the body. It will return to the Found position when the hole is passed.

A hole or depression indicates a previous injury, current physical problem, a problem in its nascent stages, astral influence, or astral possession.

You can heal and balance the person's auric field using several methods:

1. Using your pendulum or L-rod, ask your higher self to make beneficial corrections in the person's energy field, as you learned to do on page 249.

2. Pray to heal the energy field by using one of the many affirmations in Chapters 9, 10, and 11 of this book (including "Closing Holes" on page 164).

3. Use the breathing technique (on page 229) of sending prana to another person.

4. Use the following hands-on healing method: Take some deep breaths and get centered. Ask your higher self to send energy through your hands from the unlimited source of pranic energy—the divine source. Then move your hands around the outer edge of the person's energy field, packing the holes with

quick motions, as though you are packing snow onto a snow-man. Then smooth and fluff the energy field by patting the surface of the field.

Once you have supercharged the person's energy field with one of these methods, measure the auric field again and see how large and symmetrical it now is. You may be astounded.

Atmospheric Energy Fields

Master dowser Thomas Milliren[2] of Erie, Pennsylvania, reports a case of a Mr. H, who complained of serious numbness in his hands and feet, which had spread to his elbows and knees. In addition, Mr. H's severe back pain was not responding to medication. These problems began about one year after retirement.

Measuring with an L-rod, Thomas noticed the aura around Mr. H's feet, hands, lower legs, and forearms was completely missing. Thomas charged Mr. H's energy field, and his pain subsided, only to return one week later. So Thomas decided to check Mr. H's property for possible *geo-pathic fields* (injurious, noxious zones).

When he arrived on site, Thomas observed two sickly, distorted maple trees in Mr. H's front yard. With his L-rods, Thomas found that four geo-pathic lines ran right through the house, and two passed through the maple trees. One detrimental line ran right through Mr. H's TV chair and his of-fice chair. Another geopathic field bisected Mr. H's side of the bed.

One way is to deal with geopathic zones is to drive an iron rebar into the ground where the geopathic lines intersect the outer edge of the prop-erty. That is what Thomas did. He also placed a copper wire loop around the master bed.

Thomas then charged Mr. H's energy field where his aura was miss-ing, until his field was expanded and balanced all around his body. Mr. H's pains and numbness subsided and, after several treatments, his health problems completely disappeared and did not return.

Master dowser Walt Woods of Oroville, California, reports that a se-nior in high school was suffering bulimia anorexia, and she always dressed in black. He asked the girl to send him a stick-drawing of herself. Using a pendulum, Walt discovered that two-thirds of the girl's energy field was being affected by detrimental energies. He discovered a geopathic zone running right through the head of the girl's bed. Also, she was possessed by an anorexic entity.

Working daily with his pendulum, Walt took one week to make corrections until the girl's energies were normalized. At the end of the week, she washed out the black dye from her auburn hair. She began wearing pink and other colored dresses. She wore a white dress with purple trim to her prom. Soon afterward, she was married.

These stories demonstrate how atmospheric energy fields can severely impact your physical health and how they can be corrected.

Beneficial and Damaging Energies

When you enter a building, you might sense a harmonious, peaceful, uplifting, expansive ambiance, or negative, draining, chaotic sensations. A nauseous feeling may compel you to leave. You might recoil when you enter a sick person's room, filled with dis-ease. If you have ever felt such vibrations, then you are sensitive to subtle atmospheric energies.

During my travels to India and other sacred destinations, I was fortunate to visit holy temples and other sacred sites. Some temples, in continuous operation for thousands of years, radiate a most exquisite vibration of sanctity, which permanently lifts you out of mundane concerns into heavenly spheres.

Beneficial, spiritual energy vortices are found throughout the planet in religious buildings, near bodies of water, on mountains, and in spiritual vortices, such as Mount Shasta in California, the Tetons in Wyoming, the pyramids of Egypt, Machu Picchu in Peru, and thousands of other sacred sites worldwide. However, you can create powerful spiritual vibrations or vortices in your own home or work environment.

It is believed that ley lines, Hartman Grids (magnetic lines), Curry Grids, and other geometrical configurations crisscross the earth in a grid system—lines of energy forming patterns of sacred geometry.

In fact, this earth is teeming with energy—electromagnetic fields, microwaves, television and radio waves, satellite waves, cellular waves, radioactive energies, seismic activity, earthquake fractures and faults, ley line crossings, gamma rays, vortices, poisonous gases, and so forth. Also, energies in other dimensions, such as thought-forms, entities, and other environ-mental

static, surround the planet. The earth's atmosphere is buzzing with electricity and clouded with energies.

Some of these energies are damaging to our health. Those susceptible
to EMF (electromagnetic frequencies) or other destructive energies can fall
ill when living near cellular towers, high tension wires, electric power sta-
tions, and so forth. An underground water stream is often discovered below the bed of cancer victims or seriously ill patients.

Walt Woods and other master dowsers have discovered that noxious
zones are deleterious to all living things. Grass, trees, and hedges display
stunted growth or even die in the path of geopathic energy lines. An entire
line of hedge might be healthy except for one section, which, no matter
how it is cared for, simply does not grow properly. Also, paved roads or
sidewalks crack and become discolored in a pattern of detrimental lines.

Have you ever noticed such phenomena in nature? Walk around your
own neighborhood or visit a park and see whether a line runs through the
foliage or pavement.

How to Measure Earth Energies

The most useful tool for finding both beneficial and detrimental earth
energy patterns onsite is the L-rod. First, let us locate underground water
streams with L-rods. This will be easy, because electromagnetic energies in
flowing water affect your rods powerfully.

Locating Underground Streams

After completing the Warm-Up Exercises on page 236, head outside
your home with L-rods in hand. Stand on the west edge of your property. Face east. Place your L-rods in the Ready position. Tell your higher
self aloud, "Please show me when I cross an underground stream of water
running below this property." Now take a deep breath. Relax completely
and center internally. Walk forward slowly across the property until your
L-rods move to the Found position. You may or may not get a response.

After you have covered the property from west to east, then change
directions. Stand at the north edge of the property and face south. Search
again with your L-rods. If they respond, then you have located underground water. Repeat this experiment on various properties until you become comfortable locating underground water.

Locating Geopathic Zones

Now you can follow the same instructions to locate noxious energies in the property surrounding your home. Make the following request: "Please show me any geopathic lines, detrimental energies, or other noxious zones on this property."

Geopathic lines move in a particular direction. Once you locate a zone, use one L-rod and say to your higher self, "Please show me the direction of movement of this noxious zone." Your L-rod will point in the direction of the energy's movement. This is called Line of Bearing position. (See pages 99-100.) Continue in this way until you find the entry point of the geopathic energy—where it enters the property or home.

Testing the Effects of Noxious Zones

Testing whether a noxious or geopathic zone is adversely affecting a person is quite simple. With your L-rods, measure the size of the person's aura as he/she stands outside the geopathic zone. Then ask the person to stand inside the zone while you approach him/her with your L-rods. Do not enter the geopathic zone yourself, as this will skew the readings. The person's aura will shrink when inside the noxious zone, and he/she may feel dizziness or discomfort.

Remote Searches

Remote Intuitive Kinesiology, otherwise known as *map dowsing*, can be equally effective as searching onsite. Acquire or make a map of the area to be searched. This can be a sketch of a home, apartment, commercial property, lot, office building, acreage, room, or city, a person's body, or any other space that you want to search.

Place a ruler or straightedge on the left edge of the map, and swing your pendulum in Ready position. Then tell your higher self aloud, "Please show me when the straightedge crosses the [specify underground water vein, well site, noxious zone, geopathic line, harmful energy, spiritual vortex, missing object, or other target]."

Now begin to slowly slide your ruler across the map to the right. Wherever your pendulum changes its swing to Found position, then stop the ruler and draw a line on the map. Continue across the map and draw more lines wherever the pendulum indicates. Now place the ruler at the top of the map and swing the pendulum in Ready position. Follow the same directions as before. Draw more lines wherever your pendulum responds. When you are done, your target is indicated by the pattern where the lines cross. (X marks the spot!)

How to Clear Noxious Energies

You just learned how to locate geopathic zones and noxious energies. Now you may ask, "What happens when I locate one?" In this section you will learn to clear harmful energies and increase positive vibrations in any situation or location.

It goes without saying that the prayers and affirmations in Chapters 9, 10, and 11 can effectively heal and release negative psychic energies, psychic ties, entities, thought-forms, or other negative emotional energies in the target location or person.

In addition to the power of prayer, you can also use Intuitive Kinesiology to clear negative energies and increase positive ones. Here is how:

Clearing and Increasing Positions

The first step to healing negative energies with a pendulum or L-rod is to discover your Clearing position and Increasing position with each tool.

Swing your pendulum or place one L-rod in Ready position (you cannot do this with two L-rods together). Say to your higher self audibly, "Show me the Clearing position for this tool." Your pendulum or the upper wire of your L-rod will probably spin in a counterclockwise motion. Then go back to Ready position and tell your higher self audibly, "Show me the Increasing position for this tool." Usually your pendulum or L-rod will spin clockwise. If your motions are different than described, that is okay.

Clearing and Enhancing Energy Fields

Here is how to clear negative energies from any aura, energy field, house, property, location, area, or other target: Place your pendulum or L-rod in Ready position. Ask your higher self, "Can you make beneficial corrections in this [area, property, person, and so on]?" If you get a Yes response, then place your tool in Ready position and say, "Please clear the negative energies from this [area, property, person, and so on]." Your pendulum or L-rod will then move in the Clearing position. When it stops moving, this indicates the clearing is completed.

Now say to your higher self, "Please increase the positive energies of [divine light, love, joy, power, grace, fulfillment, God Consciousness, and so forth] in this [area, property, person, and so forth]." Your pendulum or L-rod will then move in the Increasing position. When the movement stops, your process is complete.

This is a simple method, but it produces profound results.

Other Treatments for Geopathic Energies

Geopathic lines or noxious zones on any home or property can be reversed with one of the time-honored techniques here, developed by master dowsers Carl Bracy of Burney, California, Joan MacFarlane of Auburn, California, or Glady McCoy of Fayetteville, Arkansas. Carl has remotely cleared radon gas from more than 250 people's houses and permanently healed those suffering from gas poisoning. He also heals pets remotely worldwide. Joan has cleared geopathic zones worldwide, on site and remotely, since 1979. Gladys has cleared adverse energies from thousands of homes, offices, and people.

Before using any of these methods, use your dowsing tool to ask your higher self which method will be most effective. Also, ask exactly where and in what direction to place magnets and other items. Once you have completed the remedy, use your L-rod or pendulum to check the person or property. Make sure the noxious energies are cleared.

1. Drive an 18-inch by 1/2-inch iron rebar vertically into the ground outside in the center of the geopathic ground-line at the entry point into the home or property. Be sure to drive the rebar deep enough so it does not get caught in a lawn mower.

2. Place blue paint, blue glass, blue surveyors flagging, or blue plastic tape at the entry point of the geopathic zone. Circle the bed's box springs with blue plastic tape. Place blue plastic tape along the edge separating the engine from the cab under the hood of the car. Blue is yin and all noxious radiations are yang, so the blue color deflects geopathic energies.

3. Place a low-gauss magnet behind the copper ground wire at the base of power poles. Place small, low-gauss magnets at both ends of power lines or anywhere that will effectively block detrimental energies from the power lines.

4. Place a copper loop in the shape of an omega symbol (Ω) at the entry point of the noxious energy. Place the loop end toward the home and the open end away from the home.

5. Place single insulated or bare #12 or #14 copper house wire around the lower edge of a bed's box spring, along a room wall, or outside a house, to block the noxious energy entry point. Do not fasten the wire together at the ends. Leave at least a 6-inch gap. Staple or tape the loose ends to a stick or board so they face each other.

6. On a map of the property, staple the place on the map where the noxious line enters the property. Or place tiny magnets on the map at the entry point. Or draw three nested omega loops with a blue marking pen to "catch" the noxious lines at their entry points. File the "healed" map in a safe place and do not dispose of it. I know this sounds fantastic, but amazingly, it works.

7. After clearing noxious energies, swing your pendulum in Ready position with one hand and hold a water faucet in the other. Ask your higher self to detoxify all harmful radiations from your energy field. Your pendulum will move in the Clearing position until these energies are removed. If your piping is plastic, then run the water as you do this.

Fascinating Energetic Discoveries

A remarkable discovery was recently made by spiritual dowser Joey Korn and his research partner, Dr. Jim Wallace, both from Augusta, Georgia.

Most aura researchers believe auric fields around human beings consist of spherical or egg-shaped energy bands. This supposition is drawn from clairvoyants' observations of layered coronas around people. Also, dowsing tools react to layered bands of energy around humans, plants, and animals when measured from any direction. It is assumed these bands form concentric circles or rings. However, Joey's research does not support this hypothesis.

By using L-rods to carefully measure the fields of energy leys, power spots, trees, plants, and human beings, Joey and Jim recognized previously undiscovered, unseen patterns of energy in the universe.

Energy leys are defined as lines of energy coursing the earth in straight lines. These intersect to create energy fields known as *power spots*. Intersecting energy leys are commonly found in sacred places, such as Stonehenge and the Great Pyramid. Human energy fields are strengthened and expanded near power spots.

When Joey and Jim meticulously mapped and marked the bands in the energy field of power spots, expecting concentric circles, they were surprised to find two interrelated spirals rather than circular or oval shapes. Joey and Jim found that the energy fields around plants, trees, animals, and human beings also form spiraling vortices.

This validated the findings of Walter Russell (1871–1963), philosopher, scientist, architect, musician, artist, author, and cofounder of the University of Science and Philosophy in Waynesboro, Virginia. Russell taught that all energy moves in vortices, made of positive/masculine and negative/feminine spiraling energy bands. Every natural vortex is charged by a positive/masculine band that spirals in centripetally, and is discharged by a negative/feminine band that spirals out centrifugally. This two-way action is also part of the whirlpool created by a flushing toilet or draining water.

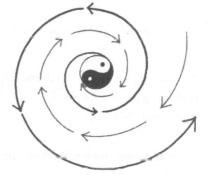

Please refer to Figure 16e, which shows a vortex with incoming positive band and outgoing negative band.

Now you can experiment. Approach a tree or a plant with L-rods and say,

Figure 16e. Energy Spirals

"Please show me an energy band in this [plant's, tree's] energy field." When your L-rods move into Found position, mark the spot on the ground. Then move slightly to the right and measure that same energy band again. Mark it. Cover up the first few marks so your previous marks do not influence your dowsing reactions. Continue to move to the right, marking the spot of each reaction. When you return to your original marks, uncover them. Do your last marks meet the first marks, or do they fall inside or outside them? If they do not meet, then the bands form a vortex, which you can validate by continuing to measure the band. If they do meet, they form a circle.[3]

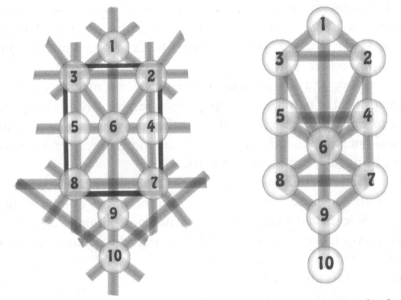

Figure 16f. Human Energy Pattern   *Figure 16g. Tree of Life*

Joey Korn discovered another amazing phenomenon with his dowsing rods: a grid pattern in the shape of the Kabbalistic Tree of Life over everyone's bed. He calls this energy matrix the Human Energy Pattern. It goes wherever you go, and you imprint it whenever you lie down on something, such as a bed. Joey calls this the Bed Pattern.

According to ancient teachings of Kabbalah, the Tree of Life was the first act of creation. God patterned everything in the universe upon this cosmic blueprint. Joey believes the Bed Pattern/Human Energy Pattern is the human soul level of the Tree of Life. Joey found that this pattern extends as a network throughout the environment and possibly the entire universe. You can see this network forming in Figure 16f on page 262. Joey calls this the Extended Human Energy Matrix.

These two figures show a comparison between the Bed Pattern and Tree of Life. The black rectangle represents the bed. The Bed Pattern consists of seven mated pairs of energy lines, or channels of energy. Imbalances in your life manifest imbalances in your Human Energy Pattern/Bed Pattern. Imbalances dowse as detrimental or noxious energy lines. Balanced energies dowse as beneficial. Because your Bed Pattern reflects your Human Energy Pattern, you can check your own imbalances around your bed with your L-rods or pendulum, by saying, "Please show me any detrimental energy lines in my Bed Pattern."

Almost everyone has some imbalances in their patterns. This is because reactions to life issues cloud the channels in energy patterns. Once you find your imbalances, you can transform them to beneficial and balance them through prayer, making these energy lines beneficial. Balancing your energy patterns helps resolve issues and heal conditions related to these imbalances.

Here is Joey's blessing to keep your Bed Pattern and Human Energy Pattern balanced. You can adapt it to include a companion that you may be sleeping with. Say this blessing while facing your bed:

Dear God, if it be Thy Will,
May the Powers of Nature converge
To increase and enhance the beneficial energies
And balance any detrimental energies
Within my (our) being(s)
And in my (our) living environment,
Especially here around the bed,
To bring healing and balance
To my (our) complete being(s):
Physically, emotionally, mentally, and spiritually.
Work especially with the Bed Pattern
And the Human Energy Pattern,
And help me (us) resolve issues
Related to imbalances in my (our) pattern(s)
For now and into the future,
For as long as is appropriate.
Amen.

Learn more about Joey Korn's work and get his books, *Dowsing: A Path to Enlightenment* and *The Secret of the Tree of Life,* at *www.dowsers.com.* You can e-mail him at *Joey@dowsers.com.*

You are filled and surrounded by a wonderful, invisible world of subtle energies. You can learn to explore, "see," and work with this fascinating world using the tools you have learned about in this chapter.

Next, in the final chapter, you will practice a profound, energizing, and spiritually lifting meditation specifically designed to lift and expand your aura.

17

Using Deep Meditation

∞

Transforming Your Energy Field

"Let the light penetrate the darkness until the darkness shines
and there is no longer any division between the two."
—Hebrew proverb[1]

Practicing meditation is the most profound way to increase the vibrational frequency in your auric field and thereby transform your life. In this chapter you will practice a powerful meditation that can cleanse, heal, purify, and strengthen your energy field. This is a guided deep meditation, practiced by following the instructions here.

I recommend that you read the meditation aloud very slowly, gently, and softly while you record it onto your computer as an mp3 file or burn a CD. Then your own voice will guide you into deep meditation. Or you can order a guided meditation CD at *www.divinerevelation.org*.

You can meditate sitting in a chair, couch, bed, or any other comfortable place. The most important instructions for this meditation are:

1. Be comfortable.
2. Do not strain or exert any effort.
3. Let go and do nothing except follow the instructions.

When breathing colors, imagine each color streaming from a divine light above your head and then flowing downward to completely saturate your energy field. All other details about meditation can be found in my books *Exploring Meditation, How to Hear the Voice of God*, and *Divine Revelation*.

Aura Meditation

Let there be light. The loving, empowering, healing, Bless-ed white fire of the Holy Spirit, in and through this healing aura meditation now, for the highest good of myself, and all others concerned.

Let there be light. The loving, empowering, healing, Bless-ed golden sphere of protective light of Jesus, in and through this healing aura meditation now, for the highest good of myself, and all others concerned.

Let there be light. The loving, empowering, healing, Bless-ed protective blue flame sword of truth of Archangel Michael, in and through this healing aura meditation now, for the highest good of myself, and all others concerned.

Let there be light. The loving, empowering, healing, Bless-ed pink, gentle, soft light of Mother Mary and Quan Yin, in and through this healing aura meditation now, for the highest good of myself, and all others concerned.

Let there be light. The loving, empowering, healing, Bless-ed violet cleansing flame of Saint Germain, in and through this healing aura meditation now, for the highest good of myself, and all others concerned.

Let there be light. The loving, empowering, healing, Bless-ed clear light of enlightenment of Mahavatar Babaji, in and through this healing aura meditation now, for the highest good of myself, and all others concerned.

I call upon the heavenly hosts, the angels and archangels of the seven rays, and all the beautiful many beings of light to lift my vibration into the light of God's love and truth.

The light of God surrounds me. The love of God enfolds me. The power of God protects me. The presence of God watches over me. Wherever I AM, God is, and all is well.

I now take a deep breath and go deep within.

I now let go of all cares and concerns of the day. I allow my body to settle down to deep relaxation. I now breathe a green colored light, which saturates all areas of the body, and I let go of all tension... I now release tension from my eyes...my eyebrows...the space between my eyebrows...my temples...jaw...neck...and shoulders.

I take a deep breath of blue light and go deeper. I let the shoulders drop and let go. I let go of my back...upper back...lower back...chest... and stomach. I let my stomach and chest drop completely. I let go and relax my arms...hands...legs...feet, and whole body.

I take a deep breath of violet light and relax. I relax my entire body and settle down to deep relaxation. Peace, peace, be still. Be still and be at peace.

I now allow my awareness to expand from this physical body to my higher bodies that surround this physical form. I now become aware of my vital body, which surrounds and permeates this body. I now breathe a vital red light of prana into the vital body. This vital body of radiant light is filled with pranic energy, coursing through my nadis and chakras, bringing life energy to every nerve and cell.

I now take a deep breath and go deeper.

I now become aware of my mental/emotional body, with permeates and surrounds my vital body. This body, of multicolored light, now settles down to inner peace and quietude, as I breathe a soft orange light into this body. I now let go as my mind becomes peaceful, still, and serene, like a still pond, without a ripple. My mind is quiet, still, radiant, and relaxed, in perfect peace.

I now take a deep breath and go deeper.

I now become aware of my intellect body. As I breathe a gentle yellow light into this body, I move through any ego-barriers that have separated me from the divine light of God's love.

I now take a deep breath and go even deeper. I now walk through the seeming façade body or veil that has separated me from my true nature of being, from my own higher self. I now break through the seeming wall of illusion, which has held me in bondage.

I now take a deep breath and go even deeper, as I walk through the gate into Spirit. I take another deep breath and completely let go.

I now become aware of my blissful body, as I meet my etheric soul self, my immortal divine soul, which vibrates with multi-colored, radiant light. It is ever-youthful and effervescent with divine love. I now breathe a rainbow of divine light in and through my energy field.

I now open to receive the blessings of my Christ-self body, filled with radiant golden light. This body may surround, fill, or hover above my physical body. I now breathe this pure, scintillating, shining gold light into my energy field.

I AM now aware of my "I AM" self body, which is filled with beautiful silver light of radiance and glory. This body encompasses my physical form and fills it with brilliance. I now breathe clear, radiant silver light into my energy field.

I now open to my God-self body, of pure white light. I open my heart to God's love, and I allow God's radiance to pour into my being. As I turn my face to God, the heavenly light of God's love pours into my being. The streams of God's light vibrate and radiate around me. I am filled with God's beauteous light of love. God's divine light fills my energy field with beauty and grace. I surrender to the divine light of God's love, and I bathe in the glory of God's radiance. I now breathe pure white light into my entire energy field. I unify with this loving presence of God.

I AM the love that God is. I AM the light that God is. I AM the power that God is. I AM the strength that God is. I AM the glory that God is.

I now take a deep breath and go deeper.

My energy body now expands to encompass the entire universe, as I become aware of my cosmic-self body. This body is large, vast, and profound. It vibrates throughout the entire creation with galactic light, divine radiance, and cosmic glory. My body is filled with cosmic life, and all the stars, the galaxies, and the Milky Way course through my body. I now breathe the breath of cosmic life into my being.

I now expand further, beyond the boundaries of the cosmic body. I now experience my absolute body, which is nameless, formless, absolute, limitless, boundless, and beyond all relative conditions. This is the experience of pure silence, deep abiding peace, the all-powerful, all- seeing, all-knowing eternal life. I now breathe the clear light of enlightenment into my being.

I AM beyond the boundaries of duality. I AM oneness. I AM wholeness. I AM the perfection of being. I AM perfection everywhere now. I AM That. Thou are That. All this is That. That alone is.

I now take a deep breath and merge completely into the oneness and sit in complete silence for a few minutes.

I now thank God for this meditation and all the profound experiences I have received. I begin to come forth from this meditation slowly, as I take some deep, vigorous breaths and pretend I am blowing out candles. As I slowly become aware of my own individuality, I "blow out" some candles. As I notice the feeling in my body, I blow out more candles. As I stretch and feel my body moving, I blow out more candles. As I become aware of my environment and the air and sounds around me, I blow out more candles. Once I feel that I am back, I open my eyes slowly.

Now I say aloud, in a clear voice:

"I AM awake. I AM very awake. I AM alert. I AM very alert. I AM inwardly and outwardly balanced. I AM in control. I AM the only authority in my life. I AM divinely protected by the light of my being. I close off my aura and body of light to all but my own God-self. Thank you God, and SO IT IS."

Epilogue

ལྦ

Your auric field is a wondrous place of divine light, love, power, radiance and energy. Enjoy exploring and visiting the wonders of this multidimensional, colorful place of divine light daily. Use the many techniques offered by this book to transform, purify, enrich, strengthen, expand, and augment your auric field. Your life will be filled with miracles as you discover what a radiant, powerful, divine light-being you truly are. You have my blessings on your pathway, dear radiant beam of light. Go forth and radiate the light of life, the light of divine energy. Bless everyone with your light. Be at peace.

—Holy Spirit

Notes

ಇಲ

Chapter 1

1. Zubko, 1996, 298.

Chapter 2

1. Zubko, 1996.
2. Genesis 2:7.
3. Svatmarama, 2:3.
4. Luke 8:47.
5. Luke 6:19.
6. Acts 5:15.

Chapter 3

1. *Taittiriya Upanishad*, 2:8:15.
2. *Williamjames.com*.
3. *Discover* magazine, Feb. 1988.
4. Brinkley, 1995.
5. I Corinthians 15:40.
6. I Corinthians 15:44.
7. Holmes, *The Science of Mind*, section 4, chapter 23.

Chapter 4

1. Zubko, 1996, 299.
2. Hartmann, 1891.
3. MacDougall, 1907.
4. Niedowski, 2004.
5. *Svpvril.com*.
6. Ibid.
7. Mann, 1973.
8. *Educate-yourself.org*.

9. Ibid.

10. Tansley, 1972.

11. Drown, *Radio-Vision*, 1960.

12. Burr, 1972.

13. Zimmerman, 1990.

14. Seto et al., 1992; Sisken and Walder, 1995.

15. Green, 1993; Tiller, 1995.

16. Becker, 1985.

17. *Biomindsuperpowers.com, spiritual.com.au.*

18. Sancier, 1996; Lin and Jiang, 1996.

19. *Totse.com/en/fringe/fringe_science/psienergybiop.*

20. *Angelfire.com/or/mctrl/ebon.htm.*

21. Ruth and Popp, 1976; Popp, 1978: *lifescientists.de.*

22. Rattenmeyer, Popp, and Nagl, 1981: *lifescientists.de.*

23. Popp and Li, 1993: *lifescientists.de*

24. Popp, Chang, Gu, and Ho, 1994: *lifescientists.de.*

25. Cohen and Popp, 1997: *lifescientists.de.*

26. Ronliang: *Journaloftheoretics.com.*

27. Alvino, 1996.

28. Rubik, 2000: *emergentmind.org.*

29. Nakamara, 2000.

30. Homestead.com.

31. Slawinski, 1987.

32. Benford, 1999: *Journaloftheoretics.com.*

33. Beal, 1996.

34. Oschman, 1997.

35. Strömberg, 1940.

36. Hall, 1969.

37. Sommer, 1969.

38. Hall, 1969.

39. *Scientific Research*, 639.

40. Bohm, 1987, 88.

41. Sheldrake, *A New Science,* 1995.

42. Sheldrake, 2002.

43. Sheldrake, 2003.

Chapter 5

1. Zubko, 1996, 300.

2. Bagnall, 1970.

Chapter 6

1. Zubko, 1996, 300.

2. Nielsen, 1977, 14.

3. Einstein: *dowsingworks.com.*

Chapter 7

1. Zubko, 1996, 298.
2. Pierrakos, 1971.
3. Hunt, 1995.
4. Cayce, 1945, 10.
5. Ibid, 5.

Chapter 8

1. Zubko, 1996, 298.
2. Maretha, 1986.
3. Genesis 37:3–50:26.
4. Genesis 1:3.
5. Luke 10:27.

Chapter 9

1. Zubko, 1996, 300.
2. *Washington Post,* Sept. 30, 1988.
3. *The Oprah Winfrey Show,* 11/15/04.
4. Contact Gladys McCoy at *www.ozarkresearch.org.*
5. *www.ozarkresearch.org.*

Chapter 10

1. Zubko, 1996, 299.
2. More information at *www.divinemotheronline.net.*
3. ©2004, text and methodology, Divine Mother's Vibrational Tools.
4. Ibid.
5. Ibid.

Chapter 11

1. Zubko, 1996, 299.
2. Cayce, 1945, 9.

Chapter 12

1. Zubko, 1996, 300.
2. © 2004, text and methodology, Divine Mother's Vibrational Tools.
3. Ibid.
4. Ibid.
5. Ibid.
6. Ibid.
7. © For more information about Connie Huebner and Divine Mother's Vibrational Tools, contact the Center at 409 W. Broadway, Fairfield, IA 52556, phone (641) 472–0662.

Chapter 13

1. Zubko, 1996, 298.
2. Panchadasi, 1940.
3. Colville, 1970, 27.
4. Jones, 1982, 111.
5. Exodus 26:1.
6. Numbers 4:6.
7. Esther 8:15.
8. Jones, 1982, 114.
9. Colville, 1970, 27.
10. Ibid.
11. Jones, 1982, 117.
12. Colville, 1970, 43.

Chapter 14

1. Zubko, 1996, 298.

Chapter 15

1. Zubko, 1996, 300.
2. Dennison, *Brain Gym Teacher's Edition*, 25.
3. Dennison, *Brain Gym for Business*, 35.
4. Dennison, *Brain Gym Teachers Edition*, 32.
5. Dennison, *Brain Gym for Business*, 51.
6. Dennison, *Brain Gym Teachers Edition*, 5.
7. Dennison, *Brain Gym for Business*, 48.
8. Dennison, *Brain Gym Teachers Edition*, 4.
9. Dennison, *Brain Gym for Business*, 37.
10. Dennison, *Brain Gym Teachers Edition*, 31.
11. Dennison, *Brain Gym for Business*, 46 and 47.

Chapter 16

1. Zubko, 1996, 299.
2. Millerin, 1988.
3. Adapted from Joey's book, *Dowsing: A Path to Enlightenment,* and from his Website at *www.dowsers.com.*

Chapter 17

1. Zubko, 1996, 300.

Bibliography

ುಂಲ

Books, Periodicals, and Television

Alvarado, Carlos S. "Concepts of Force in Early Psychical Research." *Proceedings of Presented Papers: The Parapsychological Association 44th Annual Convention* (2001): 9–24.

Alvino, Gloria. "The human energy field in relation to science, consciousness and health." *21st Link* (February 1996).

Amber, R. B. *Color Therapy: Healing with Color.* New York: Aurora Press, 1983.

Anderson, Mary. *Colour Healing: Chromotherapy and How it Works.* Bungray, Suffolk, UK: Richard Clay, 1979.

Andrews, Ted. *How to See and Read the Aura.* St. Paul, Minn.: Llewellyn Publications, 1991.

Bagnall, Oscar. *The Origins and Properties of the Human Aura.* New York: University Books, 1970.

Beal, J. B. "Biosystems liquid crystals and potential effects of natural and artificial electromagnetic fields (EMFs)." *Second Annual Advanced Water Sciences Symposium,* Exploratory Session 1, Dallas, TX (1996).

Becker, Robert, and Gary Selden. *The Body Electric: Electromagnetism and the Foundation of Life.* New York: William Morrow and Company, Inc., 1985.

Bohm, David, and F. David Peat. *Science, Order and Creativity.* New York: Bantam Books, 1987.

Brennan, Barbara Ann. *Hands of Light—A Guide to Healing Through the Human Energy Field.* New York: Bantam Books, 1988.

Brinkley, Dannion. *Saved by the Light.* New York: HarperTorch, 1995.

Burr, Harold Saxton. *Blueprint for Immortality: The Electric Patterns of Life.* London: Neville Spearman, 1972.

Cayce, Edgar. *Auras: An Essay On The Meaning of Colors.* Virginia Beach, Va.: A.R.E. Press, 1945.

Clark, Linda A. *The Ancient Art of Color Therapy.* Old Greenwich, Conn.: The Devin-Adair Company, 1975.

Colville, W. J. *The Human Aura and the Significance of Color.* Mokelumne Hill, Calif.: Health Research, 1970.

Dennison, Paul E., Ph.D., and Gail E. Dennison. *Brain Gym: Teacher's Edition Revised.*
     Ventura, Calif.: Edu-Kinesthetics, Inc., 1989.
Dennison, Paul E., Ph.D., Gail E. Dennison and Jerry Teplitz. *Brain Gym for Business.*
     Ventura, Calif.: Edu-Kinesthetics, Inc., 1994.
Dinshah, Darius. *Let There Be Light—Practical Manual for Spectro-Chrome Therapy.*
     Malaga, N.J.: Dinshah Health Society, 1996.
Discover. New York: Discover, February, 1998.
Drown, Ruth. B. *Radio Vision: Scientific Milestone.* Hollywood, CA: Drown
     Laboratories, 1960.
Eddy, Mary Baker. *Science and Health with Key to the Scriptures.* Boston: Writings of
     Mary Baker Eddy, 1994.
Green, Elmer E., P. A. Parks, P. M. Guyer, S. L. Fahrion, and L. Coyne, "Anomalous
     Electrostatic Phenomena in Exceptional Subjects." *Subtle Energies* 2 (1993): 69.
Hall, E. T. *The Hidden Dimension.* New York: Doubleday, 1969.
Hartmann, Frantz. *The Life and The Doctrines of Paracelsus.* New York: John W. Lowell
     Co., 1891.
Holmes, Ernest. *The Science of Mind.* New York: Dodd, Mead and Co., 1938.
     Holy Bible. Iowa Falls, Iowa: World Bible Publishers.
Hunt, Valerie. *Infinite Mind: The Science of Human Vibrations.* Malibu, Calif.: Malibu
     Publishing Co., 1995.
Jones, Alex. *Seven Mansions of Color.* Marina del Rey, Calif.: DeVorss & Co., 1982.
Kilner, Walter J. *Human Atmosphere, or the Aura Made Visible by the Aid of Chemical
     Screens.* New York: Samuel Weiser, Inc., 1973.
Korn, Joseph. *Dowsing: A Path to Enlightenment.* Augusta, Ga.: Kornucopia Press, 1998.
Lewis, H. Spencer. *Color—Its Mystical Influence.* San Jose, Calif.: Rosicrucian Supply
     Bureau, 1950.
Lin, H., and H. Yan Xin Jiang. "Qigong, science and practice." *21st Link* (1996).
MacDougall, Duncan, M.D. "Hypothesis Concerning Soul Substance Together with
     Experimental Evidence of The Existence of Such Substance." *American
     Medicine* (April 1907).
Mann, W. E. *Orgone, Reich and Eros.* New York: Simon and Schuster, 1973.
Maretha. *The Aura As I See It.* Self-published, 1986.
Mermet, Abbé. *Principles and Practice of Radiesthesia.* London: Stuart & Watkins, 1967.
Millerin, Thomas. *Ancient Mysteries of Healing.* Erie, Penn.: Thomas Millerin, 1988.
Millerin, Thomas J., Karen Troiani, ed. *Noxious (Geopathic) Fields Are Damaging to Your
     Health.* Erie, Penn.: Thomas Millerin, 1997.
Moss, Thelma, and John Hubacher, *The "Phantom Leaf Effect" As Revealed Through
     Kirlian Photography.* Los Angeles: UCLA Center for the Health Sciences, 1974.
Motoyama, Hiroshi. *The Correlation Between Psi Energy And Ki.* Tokyo: Human Science
     Press, 1991.
Nakamura, H., H. Kokubo, D. Parkhomtchouk, W. Chen, M. Tanaka, T. Zhang, T.
     Kokado, M. Yamamoto, and Fukuda, N. "Biophoton and temperature changes
     of human hand during Qigong." *Journal of ISIS* 18:2 (September 2000).

Niedowski, Erika. "How much does a human soul weigh? At least one scientist tried to find the answer." *Baltimore Sun* (February 2, 2004).

Nielsen, Greg, and Joseph Polansky. *Pendulum Power.* Rochester, Vt.: Destiny Books, 1977.

Oldham, G. R. "Effects of changes in workspace partitions and spatial density on employee reactions: A quasi-experiment." *Journal of Applied Psychology* 73 (1988): 253–258.

Oprah Winfrey Show, The. November 15, 2004.

Oschman, J. L. "What is healing energy?" *Journal of Bodywork and Movement Therapies* 1:3 (1997): 179–194.

Ostrander, Sheila, and Lynn Schroeder. *Psychic Discoveries.* Emeryville, Calif.: Marlowe & Company, 1997.

Ouseley, S. G. J. *The Science of the Aura.* London: L. N. Fowler & Co. Ltd., 1949.

Panchadasi, Swami. *The Human Aura, Astral Color and Thought Forms.* Chicago: Yoga Publication Society, 1940.

Pierrakos, John C. *The Energy Field in Man and Nature.* New York: Institute of Bioenergetic Analysis, 1971.

Ramacharaka, Yogi. *Science of Breath.* Chicago: Yoga Publication Society, 1904.

Regush, Nicholas, ed. *The Human Aura.* New York: Berkley Publishing Corporation, 1974.

Sancier, K. "Medical Applications of Qigong." *Alternative Therapies* 2:1 (1996): 40–46.

Scientific Research on Maharishi's Transcendental Meditation and TM-Sidhi programme: Collected Papers, Volume 1. Vlodrop, Holland: Maharishi Vedic University Press, no date.

Seto A, Kusaka C, Nakazato S, et al. "Detection of extraordinary large biomagnetic field strength from human hand." *Acupuncture and Electro-Therapeutics Research International Journal* 17 (1992): 75-94.

Sheldrake, Rupert. *A New Science of Life: The Hypothesis of Morphic Resonance.* Rochester, Vt.: Inner Traditions International, 1995.

——. *Dogs That Know When Their Owners Are Coming Home: And Other Unexplained Powers of Animals.* New York: Three Rivers Press, 2000.

——. *The Presence of the Past: Morphic Resonance & the Habits of Nature.* Rochester, Vt.: Inner Traditions International, 1995.

——. *The Sense of Being Stared At: And Other Aspects of the Extended Mind.* New York: Crown, 2003.

Shumsky, Susan G. *Divine Revelation.* New York: Fireside, 1996.

——. *Exploring Meditation.* Pompton Plains, NJ: New Page Books, 2001.

——. *Exploring Chakras.* Pompton Plains, NJ: New Page Books, 2003.

——. *Exploring Auras.* Pompton Plains, NJ: New Page Books, 2005.

——. *Miracle Prayer.* Emeryville, Calif.: Celestial Arts, 2006.

——. *How to Hear the Voice of God.* Pompton Plains, NJ: New Page Books, 2008.

——. *Ascension.* Pompton Plains, NJ: New Page Books, 2010.

——. *Instant Healing.* Pompton Plains, NJ: New Page Books, 2013.

Sisken BF, Walder J. "Therapeutic aspects of electromagnetic fields for soft tissue healing." In: Blank M, ed. *Electromagnetic fields: Biological interactions and mechanisms. Advances in Chemistry Series,* 250 (1995): 277–285.

Slawinski, J. "Electromagnetic Radiation and the Afterlife." *Journal of Near-Death Studies* 6:2 (1987): 79-94.

Sommer, R. *Personal Space: The Behavioral Basis of Design.* Englewood Cliffs, N.J.: Prentice Hall, 1969.

Strömberg, Gustaf. *The Soul of the Universe.* Philadelphia: David McKay Company, 1940.

Svatmarama. Pancham Sinh, trans. *Hatha Yoga Pradipika.* Allahabad, India: Sudhindra Nath Vasu, the Panini office, Bhuvaneswari Asrama, 1914.

Tansley, David V. D.C. *Radionics and the Subtle Anatomy of Man.* Essex, England: C. W. Daniel Co., 1972.

Tiller, W. A., E. E. Green, P. A. Parks, and S. Anderson. "Toward Explaining Anomalously Large Body Voltage Surges on Exceptional Subjects: Part I, The Electrostatic Approximation." *Journal Of Scientific Exploration* 9 (1995): 331.

Von Reichenbach, Karl, and F. D. O'Byrne. *Odic Forces or Letters on Od and Magnetism.* Whitefish, Mt.: Kessinger Publishing, 2003.

Washington Post. September 30, 1988.

White, John Warren, and Stanley Krippner. *Future Science: Life Energies and the Physics of Paranormal Phenomena.* New York: Doubleday, 1977.

Zimmerman, J. "Laying-on-of-hands healing and therapeutic touch: a testable theory." *BEMI Currents, Journal of the BioElectroMagnetics Institute* 2 (1990): 8–17.

Zubko, Andy. *Treasury of Spiritual Wisdom.* San Diego, Calif.: Blue Dove Press, 1996.

Internet Sites

angelfire.com/or/mctrl/ebon.htm (Popov)

angelfire.com/mo/radioadaptive/cuttler.html (Luckey)

bartleby.com/65/dr/Driesch.html (Driesch)

bestsolu.com/sadie_technology.htm (Hunt)

biomindsuperpowers.com/Pages/SubtleEnergyActions.html (Motoyama, Green)

dcs.napier.ac.uk/~phil/all%20abstracts%20(no%20pix).doc (Sommer)

dowsingworks.com/einstein.html (Einstein)

educate-yourself.org/tjc/ruthdrownuntoldstory.shtml (Drown)

emergentmind.org/sidorov12.htm (Wallace)

energyfields.org/science/becker.html (Becker)

fdavidpeat.com/interviews/bohm.htm (Bohm)

healthy.net/bios/elmergreen/ (Green)

healthy.net/scr/interview.asp?PageType=Interview&ID=289 (Green)

heilkunst.com/natural.html (Hahnemann)

hinduism.about.com/library/weekly/aa061301d.htm (Upanishads)

homestead.com/newvistas/radiogenicmetabolism.html (Luckey)

journaloftheoretics.com/Articles/1-2/benford.html (Benford)

journaloftheoretics.com/Links/Papers/INTENT.pdf (Ronliang) *lifescientists.de/ib0200e_.htm* (Popp)

ncahf.org/articles/a-b/allopathy.html (Hahnemann)

nuhs.edu/communications/publications/humanities/Jackson.pdf (Hippocrates)

ourworld.compuserve.com/homepages/health_/seeau.htm (Chalko)

psychology.ucdavis.edu/SommerR/default.html (Sommer)

reiki.org/reikinews/ScienceMeasures.htm (Zimmerman)

sharinghealth.com/researchers/beck.html (Beck)

spiritual.com.au/articles/healing/energeticmedicine_share.htm (Motoyama)

svpvril.com/Apergy.html#TOP%20apergy (Keely)

theelementsofhealth.com/principals.htm (Hippocrates, Driesch, Helmont)

theosophy-nw.org/theosnw/science/prat-boh.htm (Bohm)

tm.org/research/summary.html (Mahesh Yogi)

totse.com/en/fringe/fringe_science/kirilia.html (Kirlian)

totse.com/en/fringe/fringe_science/psienergybiopl169520.html (Inyushin)

twm.co.nz/energ.html (Alvino)

williamjames.com/Folklore/ANATOMY.htm (Moss)

Index

ॐ

About the Author

ﬤﬤ

Dr. Susan Shumsky has dedicated her life to helping people take command of their lives in highly effective, powerful, positive ways. She is an award-winning author, foremost spirituality expert, highly acclaimed and greatly respected professional speaker, sought-after media guest, New Thought minister, and Doctor of Divinity.

Dr. Shumsky has authored *Divine Revelation,* in continuous print with Simon & Schuster since 1996, as well as many other books: *Miracle Prayer,* published by Random House; *Exploring Chakras, How to Hear the Voice of God, Ascension, Exploring Meditation, Exploring Auras, Instant Healing,* and *The Power of Chakras,* all published by New Page Books. Her books have been published in several languages worldwide, and several were number-one Amazon.com best-sellers.

Dr. Shumsky has practiced self-development disciplines since 1967. For 22 of those years she practiced deep meditation for many hours daily in the Himalayas, Swiss Alps, and other secluded areas, under the personal guidance of enlightened master from India Maharishi Mahesh Yogi, founder of Transcendental Meditation and guru of the Beatles and of Deepak Chopra. She served on Maharishi's personal staff for seven of those years in Spain, Mallorca, Austria, Italy, and Switzerland. She then studied New Thought and metaphysics for another 25 years and became a Doctor of Divinity.

Dr. Shumsky was not born with any supernormal faculties, but developed her expertise through decades of patient daily study and practice. Having walked the path herself, she can effectively guide others along their path. She has taught yoga, meditation, prayer, and intuition to thousands of students worldwide since 1970 as a true pioneer in the consciousness field. She is founder of Divine Revelation®, a unique, complete, field-proven technology for contacting the divine presence, hearing and testing the inner voice, and receiving clear divine guidance.

Dr. Shumsky travels extensively, producing and facilitating workshops, conferences, ocean cruise seminars, and tours to India, Bali, Easter Island, Machu Picchu in Peru, the pyramids of Egypt and the Yucatan, and crop circles in England; spiritual retreats and conferences in Mount Shasta, the Tetons, Sedona, the Sonoran Desert, and Santa Cruz mountains; and many other sacred destinations worldwide. She also offers teleseminars and private spiritual coaching, prayer therapy sessions, and Divine Revelation Break-through sessions.

All of Dr. Shumsky's years of research into consciousness and inner explora-tion have contributed to *The Power of Auras,* which can significantly reduce many pitfalls in a seeker's quest for inner truth and greatly shorten the time required for the pathway to Spirit.

On our Websites, *www.divinerevelation.org* and *www.divinetravels.com,* you can:

- ⚱ Join the mailing list.
- ⚱ See Dr. Shumsky's itinerary.
- ⚱ Read Chapter 1 of all of Dr. Shumsky's books.
- ⚱ Listen to dozens of free interviews and teleseminars with Dr. Shumsky.
- ⚱ Invite Dr. Shumsky to speak to your group.
- ⚱ Find Divine Revelation teachers in your area.
- ⚱ See the Divine Revelation curriculum.
- ⚱ Register for Divine Revelation retreats and Teacher Training Courses.
- ⚱ Order a CD, downloadable files, or laminated cards of healing prayers.
- ⚱ Order books, audio and video products, or home study courses.
- ⚱ Order beautiful, full-color prints of Dr. Shumsky's illustrations.
- ⚱ Register for private telephone sessions with Dr. Shumsky.
- ⚱ Register for spiritual tours, conferences, and retreats to sacred destinations.
- ⚱ Attend our free weekly prayer circles and other special live teleseminars.

When you join our mailing list at *www.divinerevelation.org,* you will receive a free, downloadable, guided mini-meditation, plus access to our free weekly telecon-ference prayer circle and our free online community group forum.

As a gift for reading this book, please use the following special discount code when you register for one of our retreats or tours at *www.divinetravels.com*: AURAS108.

We want to hear from you. Please write your personal experiences of reading and sensing auras, and of healing your energy field, your home, your office, and your relationships: email divinerevl@aol.com.